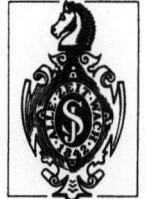

Andreas Beck

Percutaneous Transluminal Angioscopy

Forewords by E. Zeitler and W. Wenz
With 152 Figures, some in Color, and 11 Tables

Springer-Verlag
Berlin Heidelberg New York
London Paris Tokyo
Hong Kong Barcelona
Budapest

Andreas Beck M.D., Th.D.
Head of the Department of Diagnostic
Radiology and Nuclear Medicine
Klinikum Konstanz
7750 Konstanz, Germany

ISBN-13:978-3-642-74719-9   e-ISBN-13:978-3-642-74717-5
DOI: 10.1007/978-3-642-74717-5

Library of Congress Cataloging-in-Publication Data
Beck, Andreas. Percutaneous transluminal angioscopy / Andreas Beck. p.   cm.
Includes bibliographical references and index.
ISBN-13:978-3-642-74719-9 1. Angioscopy.
I. Title. [DNLM: 1. Angiography – methods. 2. Angioplasty, Transluminal –
methods. 3. Vascular Diseases – therapy.   WG500 B393p]
RC691.6.A53B431993   617.4′13059 – dc20   DNLM/DLC   92-48747

Typesetting: Mitterweger Werksatz GmbH, 6831 Plankstadt
19/3130/5 4 3 2 1 0 – Printed on acid-free paper.

For Pia, Teresa and Vincent

Foreword

"It is a real problem with abbreviations in medicine." Charles Dotter said this shortly after the first publications about techniques of and results with "PTA", which is used for "Percutaneous Transluminal Angioplasty". He gave me 26 different explanations for this abbreviation, of course not only medical ones. Now, we have got number 28: "Percutaneous Transluminal Angioscopy". I would propose to use "Vascular Endoscopy", in contrast with the surgical term "Angioscopy".

In the past few years, endoscopes with a very small outside diameter have been developed, enabling percutaneous application with frontal view. Both, the development and the application of these devices have been pushed forward considerably due to the vital interest in direct, intravital monitoring of the percutaneous procedure.

The present monography by Dr. Dr. Beck proves with its very precise photographs, that endoscopes which can be inserted percutaneously through an introducer sheath can support the exact interpretation of intravascular pathological changes.

The main problems of such interventions are the short-term interruption of the blood flow and the need for immediate infusion of water to make the vessel walls detectable.

The author contributed considerably to the solution of this problem by inserting a balloon catheter from the contra-lateral side. Manual compression and lavage with liquid complete this procedure and are, besides the excellent optics used, the basis for the high quality of the colour images.

The major advantage of angioscopy is additional information which can help to differentiate between fresh and old thrombotic occlusions. This can bring clear facts regarding the indication of aspiration, thrombolysis or mechanical treatment. Contrary to intravascular ultrasound, it does however not provide any possibility to evaluate changes within the media and adventitia.

The present studies show that following a balloon-angioplasty there mainly occur longitudinal fissures within the vessel wall which are not likely to cause a new occlusion. Different experimental investigations have proven that this fact is contributing to the good long-term results of percutaneous balloon-angioplasty, compared to surgical interventions.

Of special importance is angioscopy with a sheath for instrumentation permitting the removal of every kind of occlusion from the vascular system, under direct visualization. Further studies will help to find out for the future in which cases to apply angioscopy and when to prefer intravascular ultrasound. Under economical points of view there is much hope that the multi-directional angioscopy will help to solve most of the clinically relevant facts.

The book offers, by means of its excellent photographs detailed information on the actual state of "vascular endoscopy". I recommend it to every colleague who is interested in vascular diseases and their treatment with emphasis on control of treatment and scientific purposes.

I wish the book and its author the best of success.

Prof. Dr. EBERHARD ZEITLER
Head of Department of Diagnostics
Radiological Center
Nuremberg General-Hospital

Nuremberg, October 1992

Foreword

Shortly after percutaneous catheter angiography was introduced by Sven Seldinger in 1953 this technique became the gold standard for vascular imaging. It has been the method of choice for radiological digital substraction techniques. In recent analysis and for conventional years the improvement of clinical examination methods and the invention of color Doppler ultrasound has changed this situation. By improving Seldinger's technique angiography has become firmly established in interventional radiology and has maintained a competitive position in medicine.

In this volume my long standing coworker Dr. Andreas Beck describes a new form of vascular diagnostic procedure. After performing several thousand angiographic studies over many years, mostly for interventional procedures such as angioplasty and recanalization of vascular obstructions, he asked how it might be possible to improve the uniform angiogram and augment the analysis of stenoses and vascular occlusions. He was one of the first radiologists to have the idea of replacing the catheter by a small endoscope, an angioscope, to yield more information on the morphology of vascular stenoses and to improve the assessment of the outcome of interventional procedures.

I have encouraged Dr. Beck to pursue this challenging task, as I myself was fortunate to experience the first intraoperative experiments by Vollmar in the Surgical Department of Heidelberg University in the early 1960s. The main difference between intraoperative endoscopy and the percutaneous endoscopic technique is that the vascular lumen cannot be completely cleared of blood in the latter. Dr. Beck has overcome this problem by using simple techniques so that vascular features can be clearly visualized.

The result is a unique insight into the vascular system, on the basis of which the author has established a classification of vascular lesions. This pioneering work will be of major benefit to all vascular specialists, and I wish the book the widespread attention that it deserves.

Prof. Dr. WERNER WENZ
Head of Department of Diagnostic Radiology,
Freiburg University Hospital, FRG

Freiburg, May 1992

Preface

Until about 20 years ago radiology was the mainstay in the diagnosis and documentation of pathologic processes in the human body: in the gastrointestinal tract, the blood vessels and other organs. I still can remember the intense resistance to the new endoscopic procedures of gastroscopy and coloscopy, which posed a number of problems to radiology that we could not solve. The endoscopic pictures, however, were fascinating, as they offered the aspect of directness to diagnosis, in contrast to the indirectness of radiologic diagnosis. So, the advantages for the patient were evident, and endoscopic methods started to expand steadily.

When I asked the manufacturers of endoscopes 12 years ago if it were possible to produce endoscopes with a diameter of less than 1 mm for the examination of blood vessels, I usually met with disbelief. It was still very unusual then to substitute or supplement the standard angiographic diagnostic tools with angioendoscopy. Nevertheless, I received prototypes of different angioendoscopes from several companies, such as Olympus, Guerbet and Krauth and others with which images of widely varying quality could be achieved. There were immense problems with the first angioendoscopes, including the basic problem of receiving a reasonable image in a vessel which is always filled with blood, the lack of brightness, the lack of a documentation system, and the difficulty in handling such thin instruments and the initially imprecise interpretation of the resulting images. The real challenge of this work, though, was that of treading on new territory, viewing the inside of the vessels of a living human being.

It has never been my intention to replace angiography. I believe, however, in the high academic value of being able to verify diseases in vivo by direct vision, and previously this was only possible by indirect radiologic means.

First of all, I want to thank my honored teacher, Prof. Dr. Werner Wenz, who himself is a passionate angiographer. He did not just tolerate the experiment, which initially seemed impossible, but supported it with his advice and actions. I would also like to express my gratitude to my dear colleagues in the Departments of Radiology and

Angiology of the University Hospital in Freiburg, who always offered sound advice about performing angioscopy and in interpreting the results, often a long and cumbersome task.

A. Beck

Freiburg

Contents

1 Introduction

The first percutaneous transluminal angioplasty (PTA) was performed by Dotter and Judkins in 1964 [128]. Since then this technique has become a major interventional procedure in medicine. Over the past 8 years 4750 patients have undergone PTA at Freiburg University Hospital and Hochrhein Hospital in Bad Säckingen. A critical evaluation of complications and long-term results of this method have been reported based on this research [10, 13, 22]. Despite these long-standing experiences with this primarily angiographic method it is difficult in some patients to determine the definitive extension of the vascular disease from the angiographic radiograph and to decide whether to perform PTA. The starting point for the introduction of angioscopy was the question of whether endoscopy could add essentially new information to routine radiological investigations, and whether it was of any help in vascular interventional procedures. It was asked whether angioscopy could help in finding new criteria for pathological vascular processes that would improve the assessment of prognosis and thereby improve the assessment of prognosis and thereby improve therapeutic management of the patient.

Newer noninvasive methods of vascular diagnosis such as pressure monitoring by Doppler ultrasound and angiodynography have quickly proven themselves important in diagnosis and decision making for the angiologist. But even these procedures sometimes leave open questions regarding diagnosis and further therapeutic management [15, 16, 72]. In addition, in a number of patients PTA is difficult to perform. Its use is limited by the technically inadequate material of the guide wires and catheters, the difficulty in passing some intravascular obstructions, and unexpected complications such as local thrombosis [61, 64, 135, 141, 147, 162]. Very rarely, allergic reactions to contrast media are a contraindication to angiography and PTA.

In these situations such a direct vascular diagnostic procedure as angioscopy is very desirable. As a number of articles have reported [7, 17, 20, 21, 42, 45, 57, 59, 109, 116], however, there are various technical difficulties. In particular, the large diameter of the endoscope ruled out transfemoral insertion, and the problem of emptying the vascular lumen of blood for visualizing the vascular wall had not been solved. We addressed these problems in our study and report here the results of our work to overcome these difficulties and make angioscopy possible.

We collaborated in the successful production of ultrathin endoscopes with an outside diameter of under 2 mm and developed a procedure to clear the vascular lumen of blood. For the first time this made angioscopy possible as an additional radiological method for vascular imaging simply by transfemoral nonoperative approach of the vessel. First, however, this procedure had to be evaluated in animal experiments before it could be used in humans [94]. Later, primary vascular diagnosis and interventional techniques were compared by angiography and angioscopy in 520 patients. Furthermore, a vascular endoprosthesis was invented, which has been used for residual vascular stenoses after repeatedly unsuccessful angioplasty. This device was also clinically evaluated by means of conventional angiography and angioscopy. Additionally, we developed a novel therapeutic concept of mechanical thrombus extraction to solve the problem of local thromboses especially of those that are not or only incompletely dissolved by local or systemic thrombolysis. This mechanical thrombus extraction device was eventually used successfully in humans. The results of dilatation, local thrombolysis, stent implantation and mechanical thrombus extraction have been compared by angioscopy and angiography. Both the implantation of stents and the method of mechanical thrombus extraction are innovations in the field of interventional angiography.

This book should be useful and of value to all physicians caring for patients suffering from vascular occlusive disease. The most important aim of this book was to offer new points of view in diagnosis and therapy of vascular diseases by direct in vivo inspection of the vascular lesions, which could be realized for the first time by percutaneous angioscopy. Generally the angioscopic information about vascular diseases will help to understand unclear clinical or angiographic diagnoses and can explain the mechanisms of the different interventional procedures.

I want to thank Prof. Dr. Werner Wenz and my colleagues of the Department of the Diagnostic Radiology in the University of Freiburg and Konstanz who gave me the opportunity to elaborate this study with their continuous excellent help and collaboration.

The angioscopical pictures in this book had been realized by the use of many prototypes and commercially available instruments (Olympus Optical, Guerbet France, Krauth, Germany).

I want to thank these companies for their help and collaboration. Without the technical support of these industries in the development of the new micro-endoscopic instruments this study would not be realized.

I thank very much to my dear colleague Dr. Martin Halle for his help in translation of this book.

2 A Historical View

2.1 History of Angiography

The history of angiography began soon after W. C. Röntgen discovered X-rays in November 1895. By the beginning of the following year E. Haschek and O. T. Lindenthal had published a report on the practical use of X-rays [182]. These two scientists showed that vessels could be made visible by contrast-producing agents. They injected a mixture of cinnabar, bismuth, and chalk (the so-called *Teichmannsche Masse*) into the brachial artery of a corpse and showed a distinct picture of the vascular system after exposure to X-rays for 1 h. At the same time they wrapped a copper wire partially around a finger for reference. They showed that X-rays were unable to pass through the metal, bone, and chalk [82, 182]. Shortly afterwards, in February 1898, the Italian U. Dutto undertook similar experiments in Rome [134]. Nonetheless, it was still a long way from these experiments in anatomical specimens and animal experiments to the first angiographic imaging in patients. In other radiological fields clinical experience had also progressed, with the use of several contrast media, including bismuth salts, in the gastroenterological tract.

In 1923 the first publications on the results of angiography in humans appeared. Two French scientists, the neurologist J. A. Sicard and the rheumatologist J. Forestier, reported on an intravascular injection of contrast medium under radiological control. They used iodized oil, later named Lipiodol, as the contrast medium. At this time only intravenous contrast investigations were performed [15, 22, 74, 87, 136, 166]. In October 1923 the pathologist J. Berberich and the physician S. Hirsch published a number of experiments using aqueous solutions of different halides [69]. For intra-arterial injection in man they first chose strontium bromide as the most effective contrasting agent (Fig. 2.1). They injected 5–10 ml of a 10% –20% strontium bromide solution into the vascular system. To prevent the rapid run-off of the contrast medium a tourniquet was applied to the patient's proximal arm. Unfortunately, the route and level of concomitant medication or anesthesia was not reported in this article. Side effects such as pain in the arm on injection of the contrast medium was occasionally noted in "sensitive" patients although the pain resolved immediately on releasing the tourniquet [69]. The first angiography of the peripheral vessels was performed with sodium iodide by B. Brooks in the United States of America in 1924 [22].

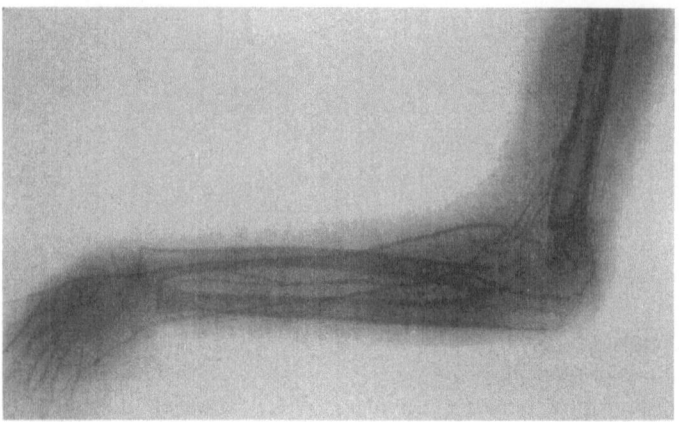

Fig. 2.1. The first angiography of a forearm (brachial artery) of a living person, performed by Beberich and Hirsch in 1923. The exposure time was 15 min

Under local anesthesia the femoral artery was surgically exposed and punctured. Angiography then followed under general anesthesia.

The door was opened for radiological imaging of intracranial vessels by the neurosurgeon E. Moniz from Lisbon, who presented his new method of arterial encephalography in Juli 1927 [280]. For contrast imaging of the cerebral arteries he initially used bromide salt solutions but later changed to sodium iodide for direct injection into the internal carotid artery. The first direct translumbar puncture of the aorta on the level of the twelfth thoracic vertebra, with subsequent imaging of the abdominal aorta and the major branching vessels by contrast medium, was performed by the Portuguese urologist dos Santos and colleagues in 1929 [322]. By the early 1950s several other publications had described modifications of the direct aortic puncture technique. This included the transcostal approach of Hoyos and del Campo in 1948 [207] and the transesophageal puncture of the aorta of Lindgren [254]. In 1948 the method of direct translumbar puncture of the aorta at the level of the 5th – 7th left intercostal space next to the vertebra was first described, a method sometimes still used today [22, 254].

Retrograde imaging of the aorta was first achieved by Ichikawa in 1938 and named "arteriography by ascending filling" [209]. A similar technique was described soon afterwards by Radner [307, 308] and Goodwin et al. [166]. They were also the first to succeed in visualizing the thoracic aorta by retrograde injection of contrast medium through a needle inserted into the surgically opened axillary artery [166, 307, 308]. A breakthrough in the technical procedure of angiography was achieved by the work of Ichikawa published in 1939 when he described a technique of advancing a urethral catheter intraoperatively from the femoral circumflex artery retrogradely up to the aorta and then injecting the contrast medium [209]. Following this report several articles about renal arteriography were published by Evans

[136], Peirce and Ramey [301] and Alken and Sommer [15] by the early 1950s.

The first percutaneous transluminal catheterization of the aorta was performed by Broden et al. in 1948 [87]; this was followed by the work of Helmworth et al. [188]. In 1953 Seldinger reported a new catheter technique, a procedure that had the greatest impact on the angiography of today. He then established and standardized this technique of vascular puncture and catheter introduction as a routine technique, and it has now become a standard procedure in angiography. This technique has therefore since been referred to as the Seldinger technique [333]. Three years later Tillander [358] and Ödman [293] for the first time performed selective angiography with hooked plastic catheters. Selective angiography of visceral arteries followed a few years later, by Biermann et al. in 1951 [74] and Wenz et al. in 1969 [398–402]. The selective catheterization of the supra-aortic arteries was reported by Voigt and Goerttler [381], Braun et al. [86], and Jönsson [219, 220] and of the coronary arteries by Conti [105].

Along with these technical innovations came improvements in the angiography equipment, which had long been inadequate. The equipment developed from the exposure of a single film to the construction of a "radiographic merry-go-round" by dos Santos, Lamas, and Caldas in 1929 [322] to Wentzlik's cassette in 1951, the simple automatic single-film changing system of Wimmer in the 1960s, the medium-sized film technique, and finally to the invention of recording by computerized subtraction angiography [22]. Examination tables are designed today to be freely mobile so that the X-ray apparatus can be moved, instead of the table with the patient, which ensures good examination of the patient from any side.

2.2 The Development of Therapeutic Angiography

Two inventions and improvements have revolutionized angiography and have led to a further increase in the number of angiographic procedures. The development, first, of therapeutic angiography resulted in a remarkable increase in the number of angiography procedures. Early experiments in interventional catheter techniques were by means of coaxial or balloon catheters for the treatment or arterial occlusive disease and by local application of fibrinolytic agents in cases of arterial thrombosis; these procedures are closely linked with the names of Dotter, Judkins [126–130], and Hess [189–191]. The second innovation was the introduction of catheter embolization techniques by Bookstein in 1974 [22], Doppmann et al. in 1968 [124], Gilsbach and Seeger [161], and Goldman et al. in 1976 [164] for embolization of benign and malignant organic or vascular lesions. These techniques have been improved and clinically used in all vascular regions, including the renal arteries [110, 149, 174, 259, 347], aorta [102, 240, 315], lower [6, 33, 142, 97, 226, 227, 238, 112, 245, 113, 261] and upper extremities

[48, 116, 171], cerebral arteries [47, 80, 114, 119, 154, 185, 221, 268, 407], visceral arteries [163], and coronary arteries [34, 12, 105].

Dotter's approach of dilating vascular stenoses by applying several coaxial catheters one within the other like a telescope [128] was replaced by Grüntzig's and Hopff's idea of using a catheter with a balloon for dilatation of the vascular lumen only at the site of the stenosis [172, 173]. In addition to the therapy of arterial occlusive disease of the pelvic and lower extremity vessels developed by Dotter and Judkins in 1964 [126–130], Dotter et al. also introduced a method of local catheter lysis in 1974 [129]. The dilatation of coronary arteries by Grüntzig and Hopff in 1974 [172] and the high-risk PTA of arteries supplying the cerebrum by Mathias et al. [268] represent the high points of conventional balloon dilatation.

2.3 Modern Interventional Techniques

After the introduction of vascular dilatation and recanalization by balloon catheter techniques several other more sophisticated techniques were developed. Laser angioplasty in man, developed by Goar et al. [162], Choy et al. [102], Geschwind et al. [159, 160], Lee et al. [247, 248], and Sanborn [320, 321], has contributed to the treatment of vascular occlusions. Thrombus extraction by catheter systems was introduced by Buxton and Mueller [92] and developed by Sniderman et al. [346] and Starck et al. [351]. The rate of reocclusion of dilated or recanalized vessels led to the construction of devices designed to keep the vessel patent. These intravascular stents were described by Cragg et al. [108, 109], and Dacie and Lumley [114], Dotter et al. [126–130], and Duprat et al. [132, 133], and were further improved by Palmaz et al. [297–299] and Urban et al. [371]. A stent that is not limited to the vascular system was designed in our department at Freiburg University and is currently on clinical trial in vascular [45, 47, 50], tracheal [60], and biliary stenosing processes [59, 62]. Stents have now been implanted on a large scale into coronary arteries by Mazieres [272] and Urban et al. [371].

Another milestone in interventional angiography has been local catheter clot lysis [21, 42, 43, 51, 58, 129, 139, 189, 190, 191], first described by Dotter et al. [129]. Very recent inventions have contributed fundamental improvements in short- and long-term results of thrombolysis. In particular, new lytic pharmacological substances such as r-TPA (tissue plasminogen activator), new transport systems for the thrombolytic agents, open guide wires, and new concepts of local lysis protocols (e.g., dose splitting) have begun to replace current lysis regimes of streptokinase and urokinase [140, 190, 226, 362].

3 Percutaneous Transluminal Angioscopy

Endoscopy with rigid instruments has been used for 40 years. The development of fiber optics revolutionized the technique and prepared the ground for its introduction into the entire medical field [316, 321]. Endoscopy had been limited largely to the gastroenterological tract and various other body cavities, but during the past few years subtle imaging of other organs that can now be reached by endoscopy has also been performed [56, 106, 137, 138]. In collaboration with our research group ultrathin endoscopes were designed 5 years ago and have opened a new dimension in diagnosis. Because of the small caliber of the new equipment angioscopy can for the first time gain ground in the field of transfemoral, nonoperative angiography, such as reaching up to the coronary arteries [99, 106, 150, 153, 247, 348, 349, 350, 356], supra-aortic branches [9, 23, 44, 54, 310], and renal arteries. First, however, the problems had to be solved of clearing the vascular lumen of blood, gaining sufficient light intensity, improving picture quality, and establishing a means of recording.

3.1 Material and Methods

3.1.1 Angioscopic Equipment

Several prototypes of angioscopes and commercially available instruments (endoscopes and recording equipment from Olympus Optical, Hamburg, FRG; Guerbet France, Krauth, Germany) are currently available measuring 0.7–2.4 mm in outside diameter with a biopsy channel of 0.1–0.35 mm (Fig. 3.1). The angioscopes are 90–120 cm long and have a similar construction to commonly used endoscopes (Fig. 3.1). The endoscope is made predominantly of a polymerized material. The lens of the endoscope, measuring 2 mm in diameter, is fixed at the tip of the endoscope by a metal mounting (Fig. 3.2). This mounting is seen well on X-ray examination, but it is relatively rigid so that this endoscope has been employed primarily in animal studies. A cold light is connected to the endoscope together with various recording devices, such as a single camera, automatic camera with winder, or a videotape recorder. Before each procedure the endoscope is gas-sterilized with a maximal temperature of 53°C, and the biopsy channel is air-dried and afterwards sterilized a second time. At short intervals bacteriological analysis is performed from a smear of the endoscope.

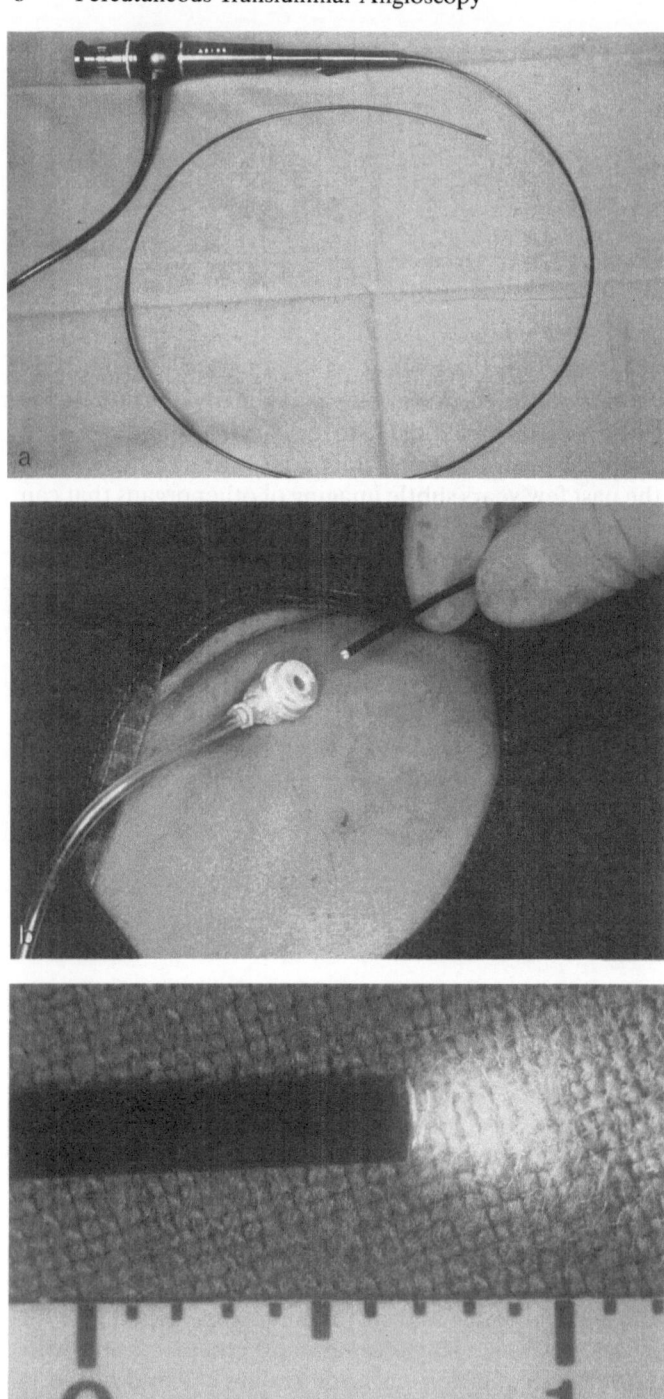

Fig. 3.1 a–c

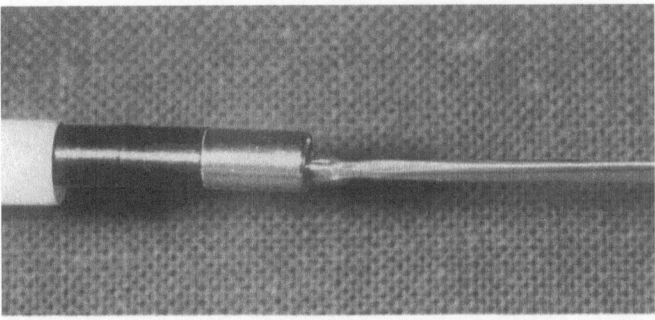

Fig. 3.2. Tip of an endoscope. Flushing with sodium chloride and probing with a wire is done simultaneously through the biopsy channel. *Left*, tip of an 8-F catheter

3.1.2 Access for Vascular Endoscopy

The access site for angioscopy is exclusively transfemoral. Under local anesthesia a 7-F introducer sheath is positioned in the vessel in the usual way. To visualize the distal femoral artery, the popliteal artery, and the trifurcation the endoscope is inserted directly through the sheath. Imaging of central vessels, such as the pelvic, renal, and supra-aortic vessels is achieved by first introducing a selective 8-F catheter through a 9-F introducer sheath under X-ray control to the region of interest. The endoscope can then be advanced through the catheter to that vascular region.

3.1.3 Intravascular Positioning of the Angioscope

The angiographic procedure of Seldinger is the basis for the vascular endoscopy technique. After puncture of the femoral artery and correct placing of the introducer sheath a thin guide wire (20–50 cm) is advanced through the dilator. The dilator is then removed before the endoscope can be advanced over the wire, which runs through the biopsy channel. The procedure of advancing the endoscope is monitored radiographically (Figs. 3.3, 3.4). Dissection of the vessel is largely avoided by this procedure; the risk does not exceed that of conventional selective angiography. If the endoscope cannot be advanced smoothly at the puncture region, the distal end of the introducer sheath, or within the vessel, or if vascular abnormalities are identified, the endoscope must be removed immediately. In obese patients angioscopy in possible only by using the retrograde procedure, since

Fig. 3.1.a Prototype of the angioscope PF 18 (Olympus Optical, Hamburg, FRG) measuring 1.8 mm in diameter with a biopsy channel of 0.2 mm. **b** Angioscope, 0.7 mm outside diameter. Sodium chloride solution is administered through the biopsy channel. On the *left* is a F 7 sheath set. **c** Angioscope, outside diameter 1.5 mm; the most commonly used instrument in peripheral vessels

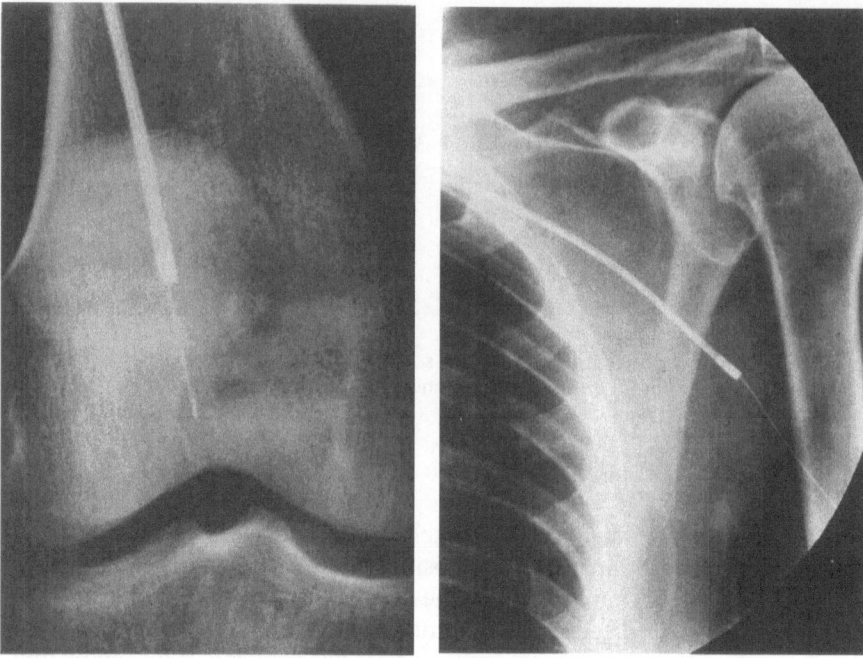

Fig. 3.3 (*left*). X-ray control of the position of the angioscope. The tip of the angioscope with guide wire is in the superficial femoral artery

Fig. 3.4 (*right*). Radiological control of the position of the angioscope. The endoscope with the guide wire is advanced to the left subclavian artery

in the antegrade puncture technique the angle between the femoral artery and the introducer sheath is relatively large so that the angioscope must be severely angulated in that area. Furthermore, angioscopy is recommended only in cooperative patients since flexing of the patient's hip bends the endoscope and may damage the optical fibers.

3.1.4 Clearing the Blood from the Vascular Lumen

The main problem in PTA is the necessity to clear the vascular lumen of blood. This problem of achieving complete emptying of the vessel is difficult, as proximal ligation or surgical opening of the vessel is not available for radiologists. Therefore, only a limited number of possibilities are available to achieve angioscopic documentation without or with only short-term reduction in the vascular blood flow.

For angioscopy of the vessels below the inguinal ligament (i.e., the distal iliac artery and femoral artery) proximal cessation of the blood flow is technically possible. A balloon catheter can be advanced from the contralateral femoral artery across the bifurcation and into the ipsilateral common

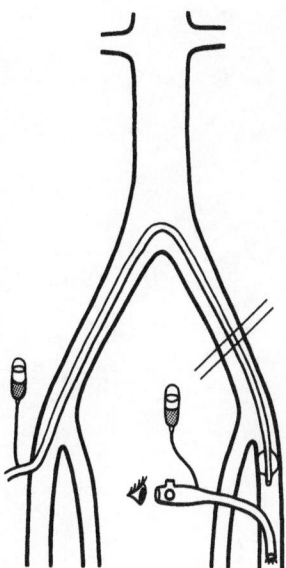

Fig. 3.5. Diagram of the procedure to empty the iliac artery by contralateral balloon catheterization and occlusion

iliac artery, where it can be inflated for the time of the angioscopic procedure (Fig. 3.5–3.9).

Puncture of the diseased side is performed with a 9-F introducer sheath in the retrograde way at the level of the inguinal ligament, approximately 4 cm distal to the blocked vascular segment. Complete blood flow reduction in the angioscopic area is not achieved by this method because extensive collateral vessels with multiple anastomoses are present in the pelvic region. The reduction in blood flow is nevertheless sufficient for angioscopic visualization, especially when a high-grade proximal stenosis is present and is further diminishing the blood flow. Despite incomplete emptying of the vessel this technique is sufficient for intravascular visualization as the residual blood is diluted and rapidly displaced by the injection of sodium chloride solution. The maximum tolerated occlusion time with this technique is 4 min.

A second possibility for reducing blood flow in the femoral and popliteal vascular system is achieved by manual compression directly above the inguinal ligament by an assistant after the femoral artery has been routinely punctured above the inguinal ligament, and a 9-F introducer sheath has been placed (Fig. 3.10). This compression is begun directly before endoscopic visualization, when the endoscope has been placed at the region of interest and the sodium chloride flush started (see Sect. 3.1.5). By this method the vascular lumen can be imaged for only a few seconds. Nevertheless, this method appears to be adequate for certain situations. This procedure is not harmful and has a low risk for the patient.

A third method for blood flow reduction is puncturing of the femoral artery above the inguinal ligament and advancing a balloon catheter approximately 10 cm in the central direction. The femoral artery is then

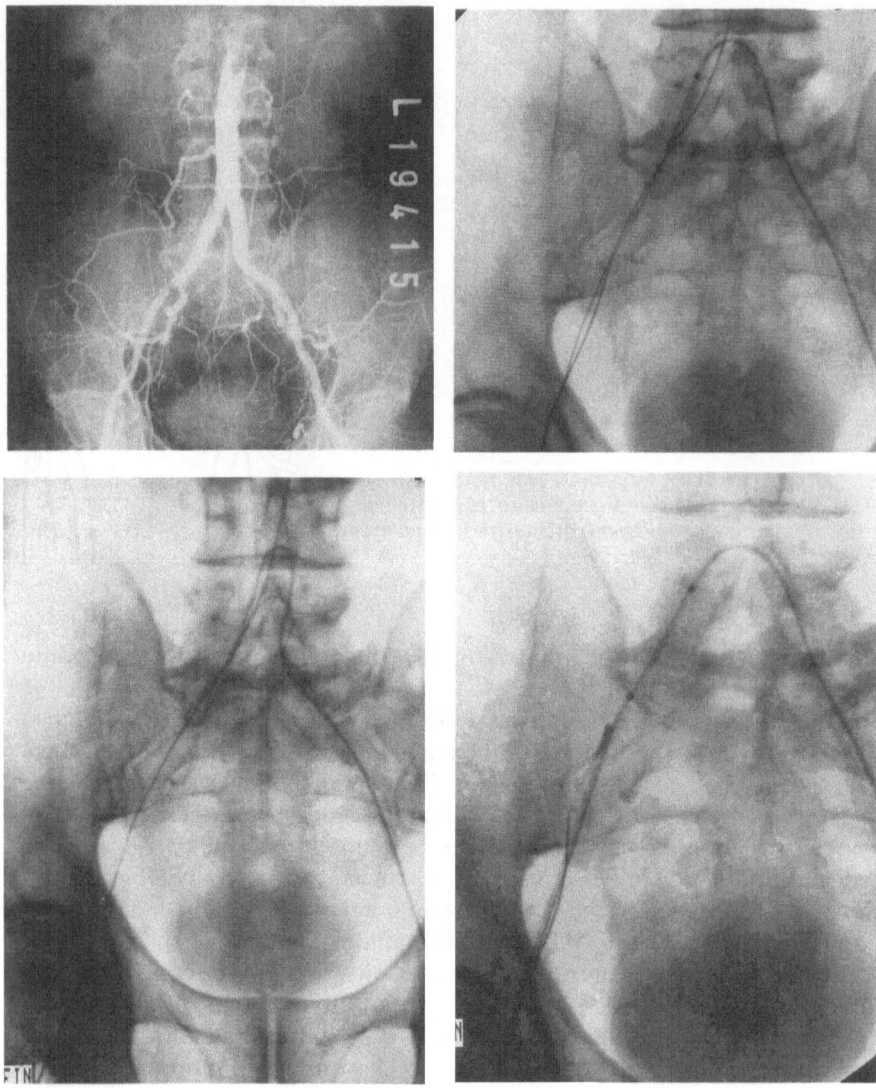

Fig. 3.6 (*upper left*). High-grade stenosis of the right external iliac artery. Catheter angiography from the left side

Fig. 3.7 (*lower left*). Catheterization of pelvic arteries from both sides

Fig. 3.8 (*upper right*). The balloon catheter is advanced from the left to the right common iliac artery

Fig. 3.9 (*lower right*). The angioscope is positioned just in front of the stenosis

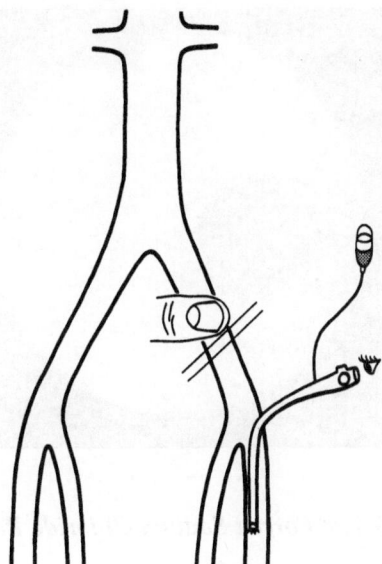

Fig. 3.10. Manual compression by an assistant of the external iliac/common femoral artery for blood flow reduction

punctured again about a hand's width below the inguinal ligament followed by the introduction of another 8-F introducer sheath. The blood flow can then be ipsilaterally blocked or at least considerably diminished for a short period of time by inflation of the proximal balloon catheter so that short-term angioscopic visualization is possible (Fig. 3.11). The indication for this procedure is extremely limited because of the insertion of two catheters in orthograde direction.

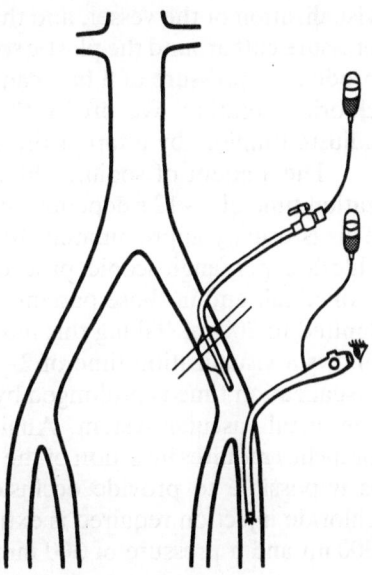

Fig. 3.11. Occlusion of blood flow by a second proximal occlusion catheter

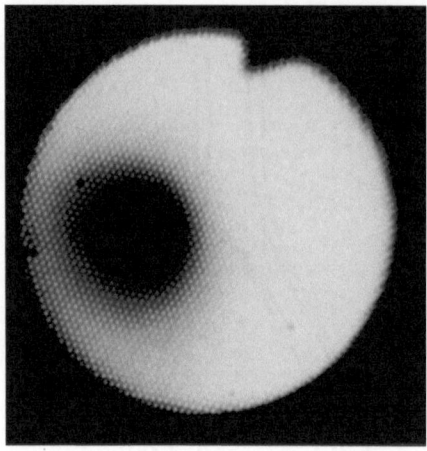

Fig. 3.12. Typical tubelike configuration of an animal artery without any change of the vascular wall (iliac artery of a dog)

3.1.5 Forced Sodium Chloride Perfusion

After occlusion of the proximal vessel, 0.9% sodium chloride solution is injected through the biopsy channel along the guide wire into the vessel. It is not mandatory to remove the guide wire from the endoscope with a diameter of 2–2.4 mm since the biopsy channel in these endoscopes is sufficiently large for both the wire and the flush solution (Fig. 3.12). If the endoscope is smaller than 2 mm in diameter, the wire must be removed prior to injection of the solution. As a consequence the endoscope can be advanced only distally under radiological control with frequent constant injection through the biopsy channel to avoid dissection of the vessel.

In general, a perfusion pressure of 250–300 mmHg is required for good visualization of the vessel, and this pressure is achieved by wrapping a blood pressure cuff around the plastic sodium chloride bottle. A roller pump, which produces a pressure of 3 bar, can also be used for administering the sodium chloride solution. We prefer the blood pressure cuff as the flow can be adjusted rapidly by a tap at the end of the infusion line.

The amount of sodium chloride solution required to achieve a visualization time of 5–12 s depends on the degree of proximal vascular occlusion. This is usually approximately 10–20 ml. A total volume of 300 ml sodium chloride per angioscopic procedure should not be exceeded in a single individual, and in those patients with a history of heart failure it should be limited to 200 ml. Taking this into account, 300 ml sodium chloride solution allows a visualization time of 2–4 min. Using the antegrade procedure the visualization time is prolonged by about 30% because of better occlusion of the distal vascular system. Angioscopy of the iliac, renal, or supra-aortic branches requires insertion of the angioscope within a guiding catheter, and it is impossible to provide occlusion of blood flow. The volume of sodium chloride injection required is extremely variable. In these cases a volume of 300 ml and a pressure of 300 mmHg should not be exceeded.

3.1.6 Recording Techniques

Since the time available for visualization of lesions by angioscopy is very limited, several photographic methods for recording the angioscopic images have been tested. Picture documentation has used a simple single-frame reflex camera with a manual winder, a reflex camera with an automatic winder and two frames per second, and a video camera with continuous monitoring (Olympus OM1; Video-Exon Camera, Olympus FV I/II Camera, Sony Umatic Recorder, Orion VHS System). The initial single-frame reflex camera was of limited value because of the slow film winding. The camera with an automatic winder provides satisfactory intravascular recording. Videotape recordings ensure immediate review of the vascular findings after the angioscopic procedure, but the resolving power of the frozen videofilm is still poor, and in view of this we prefer to use the conventional reflex cameras.

3.2 Animal Studies as a Precondition for Angioscopy in Man

In five series of experiments in dogs the procedure described in Sect. 3.1 was evaluated. In particular we tested the techniques of partial reduction or complete blocking of blood flow before their application to patients. Animals were anesthetized, the femoral artery was punctured, and a 9-F introducer sheath was positioned. After inserting the angioscope in antegrade direction, adequate view of the femoral vessel was ensured by applying the perfusing solution with a pressure of 500 mmHg. The central vessels could also be examined with the additional manual compression of the abdominal aorta.

Angioscopy of supra-aortic branches was performed with large catheters (10–13 F). When these catheters were placed at the very proximal part of the vessel, the blood flow was already diminished, and angioscopy was technically possible without any further problems. Angioscopy of the renal arteries was also studied in animal experiments. Angiography of the renal artery was performed with a 10-F selective catheter. After the tip of the catheter had been advanced very far distally into the renal artery, the guide wire was replaced by an angioscope. Since the 10-F catheter almost completely occluded the proximal lumen of the renal artery, angioscopy was possible with an infusion of 15 ml sodium chloride solution with a minimum pressure of 100 mmHg. Complications were not noted during or after the procedure in any of the five series of animal experiments. After the angioscopic procedures the animals were observed, and no late complications or other sequelae were revealed. An artery of a dog shows a totally smooth lining, and the configuration of the lumen is almost circular. Typically there are no atherosclerotic plaques or thrombotic deposits (Fig. 3.12). During angioscopy in the dogs the arteries revealed pronounced spasm which almost completely obliterated the vessel lumen. This was observed only in rare cases in man.

3.3 Indication for Angioscopy

At first only uncertain angiographic situations were indications for angioscopy. Since gaining positive experience with angioscopy in animals and reducing the diameter of the endoscopes during these experiments to sizes equal to 5-F catheters, indications for angioscopy have been continuously extended. Additionally, inspection of the angioscopic equipment by the Olympus Optical Company (Hamburg, FRG) has revealed no material fatigue or material damage that could harm the patient. The indication for angioscopy was then extended to PTA, local thrombolysis, and differentiation of local thrombosis versus thromboembolism. Another indication for angioscopy seems to be the control of angiographically impossible recanalization situations. In these cases a dissection of the vessel can be prevented by continuous angioscopic control. Direct visualization of the new interventional techniques such as intravascular stent insertion is likely to be a major field for angioscopy, and it may be especially helpful in inspection of the intimal layer within the stent. Furthermore, modern procedures of thrombus extraction with a flexible, spiral-shaped wire can be controlled impressively by angioscopy. Especially in the field of laser angioplasty angioscopy is a developing procedure, as the effects of laser angioplasty are still incompletely explained and documented in vivo. Assessment of the efficiency of electronically produced hot-tip catheters and of "microwaves" currently still on trial will be facilitated by angioscopy. The recanalization of long stenoses by the new method of rotation angioplasty could also be primarily controlled by angioscopy (Table 3.1).

Table 3.1. Current indications and diagnostic prediction of percutaneous transluminal angioscopy versus angiography

Diagnostic problem	Indication	
	Angioscopy	Angiography
Grading of atherosclerosis	++	++
Diagnosis of uncertain vascular occlusions	++	+
Differential diagnosis:		
Local thrombosis – thromboembolism	++	(+)
Inflammatory vascular changes	+	+
Actinic vascular injury	++	+
Control of PTA	++	+
Control of local lysis	++	++
Control of stents	++	+
Control of thrombus extraction	++	+
Control of rotation angioplasty	++	+

++, Unequivocal diagnostic result; +, likely diagnostic result; (+), limited diagnostic result

4 Angioscopic Diagnosis of Vascular Changes

Diagnostic criteria for PTA of vessels have not yet been defined. At present only a few research groups practice transfemoral and transluminal angioscopy in the manner described here, and consequently experience with the technique is limited. In this section angioscopic evaluation of healthy as well as atherosclerotic, inflammatory, actinic, and thrombotic changes of vessels is illustrated. It should be kept in mind that angioscopic diagnosis is at present primarily descriptive and must be assessed in relation to established angiographic criteria.

4.1 Normal Vessels

At angioscopy normal human arteries have a tubular shape with a smooth intimal surface. The vascular wall is pale pink. It can quickly be cleared of blood by flushing the angioscope with the sodium chloride solution. In contrast, this is more difficult in atherosclerotic or thrombotic vessels where blood components adhere and can only be partially removed from the vascular wall. A consistent feature of healthy vessels is their elasticity, which allows the endoscope to be advanced without resistance (Table 4.1). The blood flow returns more quickly in healthy vessels after sodium chloride perfusion compared with atherosclerotic vessels, where it is markedly prolonged. Very small vessels infiltrating the vascular wall are not normally present, but these were found in three cases with inflammatory vascular changes as well as in three patients in whom radiotherapy had damaged the vessel and caused a stenosis.

Table 4.1. Angioscopic findings of healthy human vessels

Angioscopic findings	Normal	Pathological
Tubular appearance, round or oval cross-section	+	−
Homogeneous pale pink color of all vascular parts	+	−
Vascular elasticity	+	−
Little adherence of blood components during the angioscopic flush	−	+
Quickly recurring blood stream after stopping sodium chloride flush	+	−

4.2 Pathological Vascular Features

Several pathological vascular features are observed by angioscopy: the vessels lose their tubular appearance, which is especially evident in atherosclerotic segments, but which is also present in parts of the vessel affected by inflammation or radiation. In these cases concentric or eccentric stenoses of variable degrees and complete obliteration are almost regularly observed. The most consistent angioscopic feature of pathological vascular changes are atherosclerotic plaques of different sizes and shapes. As healthy vascular endothelium is usually pale pink in color, changes in homogeneity as well as in color indicate early-stage atherosclerosis, mural thrombosis, inflammation or actinic vascular changes.

Depositions on the vascular endothelium are easily recognized by angioscopy. The degree of atherosclerosis is easily documented. Depositions can increase in size and sometimes completely cover the endothelial surface. In atherosclerotic vessels the adherence of blood components to the vascular wall is strikingly prolonged. On average twice as much sodium chloride solution is needed in atherosclerotic vessels compared to normal vessels. Frequently a permanent apposition of blood is seen in niches of atherosclerotic plaques. Clearing blood components from these vascular parts is incomplete. The characteristic elasticity of healthy vessels is markedly diminished or absent in atherosclerotic regions. Probing with a guide wire may leave traces or defects in atherosclerotic lesions. In contrast to animal arteries, these defects are recognized especially in the elderly and are well documented by angioscopy (Table 4.2).

Table 4.2. Power of representation of pathological changes in vessels diagnosed by angioscopy and angiography

	Angioscopy	Angiography
Evaluation of cross-section	++	(+)
Stenosis: eccentric-concentric	++	(+)
Inhomogeneous discoloration of vascular wall	++	−
Rigidity of the vessel	+	(+)
Atherosclerotic plaques	++	(+)
Marked prolongation of detachment of blood components	+	−
Thrombotic adhesions	++	+
Deceleration of blood flow	++	+

Diagnosis: ++, unequivocal; +, good; (+), limited; −, not possible

4.2.1 Atherosclerosis

Atherosclerotic changes of different stages can be demonstrated impressively by angioscopy (Figs. 4.1–4.16). In all atherosclerotic stages the most striking finding is discoloration of the vascular wall. In early atherosclerosis, pale pink areas are adjacent to dark pink areas that have a partly speckled (Fig. 4.1) and a partly circular striped pattern (Figs. 4.3, 4.4). In more advanced stages of atherosclerosis grayish-white plaques are predominantly found. In these stages additional vascular eccentric stenoses of different degrees are frequently observed (Fig. 4.4).

Angioscopy allows earlier detection of atherosclerotic lesions than angiography because early stages of atherosclerosis, such as an irregular vascular surface or early stenosis are not detected by angiography. The primary criterion of atherosclerosis is alteration of the vascular cross-sectional area. In our patients, 90% of atherosclerotic stenoses were caused by irregular vascular cross-sections with additional concentric or eccentric narrowing by plaques (Figs. 4.5, 4.6). In every case angioscopy revealed vascular stenosis. Angiography without radiological imaging in multiple planes had missed these findings (Table 4.3). Atherosclerotic plaques of any shape can be diagnosed by angioscopy (Figs. 4.5–4.10). Early stages of atherosclerosis show almost uniform flat depositions upon otherwise healthy endothelium whereas later stages may have any shape – at this stage eccentric stenoses are found predominantly. Radiologically concentric stenoses, often involving only one vascular segment, have been shown to be markedly more extensive and complex than previously suggested by angiography. The consistency of atherosclerotic plaques is independent of the degree of atherosclerosis. In cases of solid, flat, mural atherosclerotic plaques probing with a guide wire leaves traces, whereas eccentric and pointed plaques with

Table 4.3. Angioscopic findings in atherosclerosis

Degree of atherosclerosis
  Segmental
  Generalized

Discoloration of vascular wall
  Flat
  Circular striped
  Dusky red, grayish, white

Configuration of plaques
  Eccentric
  Concentric
  Flat
  Raised, pointed
  Raised, round
  Disseminated
  Vulnerable
  Rigid

Degree of stenosis

Configuration of stenosis
  Eccentric
  Concentric

Cross-sectional appearance

stalactite appearance are extremely firm (Figs. 4.11–4.16). The tip of these peaked plaques looks brighter than the base, which is grayish to brown-yellow in color. Figures 4.17–4.25 show the principles of aortic angioscopy and the findings of severe atherosclerosis of the aorta. Plaques of different stages are recognized, and the degree as well as the length of the stenosis is visualized well by angioscopy. In general, angioscopy has the advantage of revealing diffuse pre- and poststenotic alterations in the vascular wall that may be missed by angiography (Figs. 4.17–4.25).

4.2.2 Thrombosis

Local vascular thrombosis is technically difficult to detect by angioscopy. Because of reduced blood flow or stasis in these regions clearing the lumen with sodium chloride perfusion is delayed so that imaging of the primary lesion is not achieved in all cases (Fig. 4.26). Thrombotic deposition can be seen angioscopically only when the mixture of blood and sodium chloride solution is drained by collateral vessels, or if the residual lumen is large enough to ensure run-off of the solution. If this is not the case, permanent blurring of the view by blood components makes angioscopy difficult. If organized, local thrombosis can be localized unequivocally and thrombolysis can be initiated through the biopsy channel of the angioscope. After the tip of the angioscope has been placed directly in front of the thrombus, urokinase or streptokinase can be injected through the biopsy channel of the endoscope. Local thrombolysis can thereby be monitored and controlled under direct vision.

The surface of a thrombus has different color shades. An early thrombus, for example, is brighter than a later one, the surface of which is usually dark and may eventually become black. The character of the surface of the thrombosis is also different. Early lesions have a rough and partly fissured surface and the shape partially ascending to the side of the wall, whereas late ones usually have a retracted smooth surface which is markedly solid on guide wire probing through the endoscope. Fresh thrombotic lesions are covered by fibrinous depositions that look like floating algae when flushing with the angioscopic solution (Fig. 4.27). These fibrinous depositions stick to the vascular wall or the surface of the thrombosis. They regularly have a light red to almost white coloration. Angioscopic differences have been observed between local thrombosis and thromboembolism although both circumstances cause a reduction in blood flow in similar ways. In local thrombosis thrombotic material adheres more firmly to the vascular wall than in thromboembolism. Additionally, prolonged clearing of blood components from the vascular endothelium by angioscopic flushing is usual for local thrombosis. The light red color of the surface of the thrombotic lesion is indicative primarily of local thrombosis whereas thromboembolism characteristically has a dark to almost black appearance (Figs. 4.28, 4.29). A smooth surface of a thrombotic occlusion is indicative of a local thrombus, in contrast to the rough and fissured surface of thromboembolism

(Figs. 4.28–4.31). Intraluminal fibrin depositions that cannot be dissolved by angioscopic flush have been found primarily in local thrombosis (Table 4.4).

4.2.3 Vascular Inflammation

In three patients with primary vascular inflammatory stenoses of unknown origin angioscopy was performed at the same time as angiography. Histological analysis revealed Buergers's disease. Histologically Buerger's disease, also called thromboangiitis obliterans, can be classified into three stages. The first shows fibrinoid necrosis with leukocyte infiltration of the vascular intima and media limited to a vascular sector. The second stage is characterized by the replacement of the fibrinoid material by granulating tissue. During the third stage this granulating tissue turns into scar tissue, which is the cause for the stenosis of the vascular lumen. This disease is located primarily in the arteries of the lower extremity (juvenile gangrene of the extremities). Occasionally, central as well as renal, mesenteric, or coronary arteries are involved in addition. The first sign of the disease is fibrinoid necrosis of the intima, which favors the apposition of thrombotic material. This necrosis and thrombotic material are later replaced by granulating and connective tissue. This is followed by intimal scarring, the final stage of the disease that is often a cause for atherosclerosis (Figs. 4.32, 4.33). In comparison to atherosclerosis Buerger's disease shows distinct angioscopic features. Adherence of blood to the vascular wall when flushed with sodium chloride solution has been shown to be markedly prolonged because of the intimal scarring.

In all three cases of thromboangiitis obliterans the vascular wall appeared dusky red with cordlike connective tissue scarring of the entire wall. The finding of a "polypoid" lining of the entire vascular intima causing stenosis was very impressive. The concentric stenosis extended over the entire vascular length, in contrast to segmental stenosis in atherosclerosis. In every case of thromboangiitis obliterans the vascular changes were generalized. In

Table 4.4. Angioscopic findings of thrombotic versus thromboembolic vascular occlusion

Angioscopic findings	Thrombosis	Thromboembolism
Reduction of blood flow, stasis	+	+
Adherence of thrombotic material	++	(+)
Prolongation of detaching wall-adherent blood components	++	(+)
Color of thrombus: light red	++	(+)
Color of thrombus: dark black	(+)	++
Smooth surface of thrombus	(+)	++
Rough surface of thrombus	+	(+)
Wall-adherent fibrin depositions	++	(+)

++, Unequivocal diagnostic feature; +, diagnostic hint; (+), possible diagnostic feature

one individual vascular scarring was so severely pronounced that the usually dusky red appearance had been replaced in part by white areas. Smaller thrombotic depositions along with vascular changes were present in every patient. Examination of these patients by angioscopy has underlined the fact that the clinical manifestations of thromboangiitis obliterans, such as thrombotic vascular occlusion, are based on generalized vascular injury (Table 4.5).

Table 4.5. Summary of angioscopic features of inflammatory vascular changes

"Polypoid" internal lining of the vascular lumen
Dusky red discoloration of the luminal wall
Cordlike, white vascular scarring of the whole length
Concentric long stenosis
Additional signs of atherosclerosis
Thrombotic deposition on vascular wall
Augmented adherence of blood components to vascular wall detected by angioscopic flushing

4.2.4 Actinic Vascular Injuries

The side effects of radiotherapy of tumors are not limited to the tumor tissue but severely damage the surrounding tissue and are the cause for actinic stenoses. Four patients with actinic vascular stenoses were investigated angioscopically after a stenosis had been documented angiographically. Three of the patients had undergone radiotherapy for breast carcinoma. The stenoses were therefore all located at the branching of the subclavian artery (Figs. 4.34, 4.35). In the other individual the stenosis was located in the femoral artery because of treatment with radiotherapy of a myosarcoma in that region (Figs. 4.36, 4.37). The pathological mechanism of radiation-induced vascular stenosis is similar to the vascular changes of inflammation or thromboangiitis obliterans. Likewise, actinic vascular changes are characterized by sectorlike fibrinoid necrosis of the intima and media with leukocyte infiltration at the first stage of the disease. During the second stage the development of granulating tissue starts from the external layers and later causes intimal scarring, which may later cause the stenosis of the vessel. These changes have been observed to be accompanied by atherosclerosis.

Uniform findings of actinic vascular changes were seen at angioscopy (Figs. 4.38–4.39); in all cases extensive, flat, and disseminated scarring of the vessels of the irradiated areas with an additional augmented adherence of blood to the vascular wall was observed. Areas which had not been irradiated lacked these changes and showed only typical atherosclerotic changes. It must be pointed out that the wall of the irradiated vascular segments was more rigid and sustained compression on contact with the angioscope. A further sign of a rigid vascular structure is the lack of vascular dilatation even with high catheter balloon pressures. The appearance of actinic vascular injury is reminiscent of gastroscopic features of scarring induced by recurrent gastric ulcers. As in gastric scarring old scarring is seen next to new lesions in actinic vascular changes (Table 4.6).

Table 4.6. Summary of the angioscopic features of actinic-induced vascular changes

Scarring of different stages, scarring-induced long concentric stenoses
Wall-adherent thrombi
Rigidity of vascular wall
Scarring limited to the radiation field
Augmented wall adherence of blood components seen with angioscopic flushing

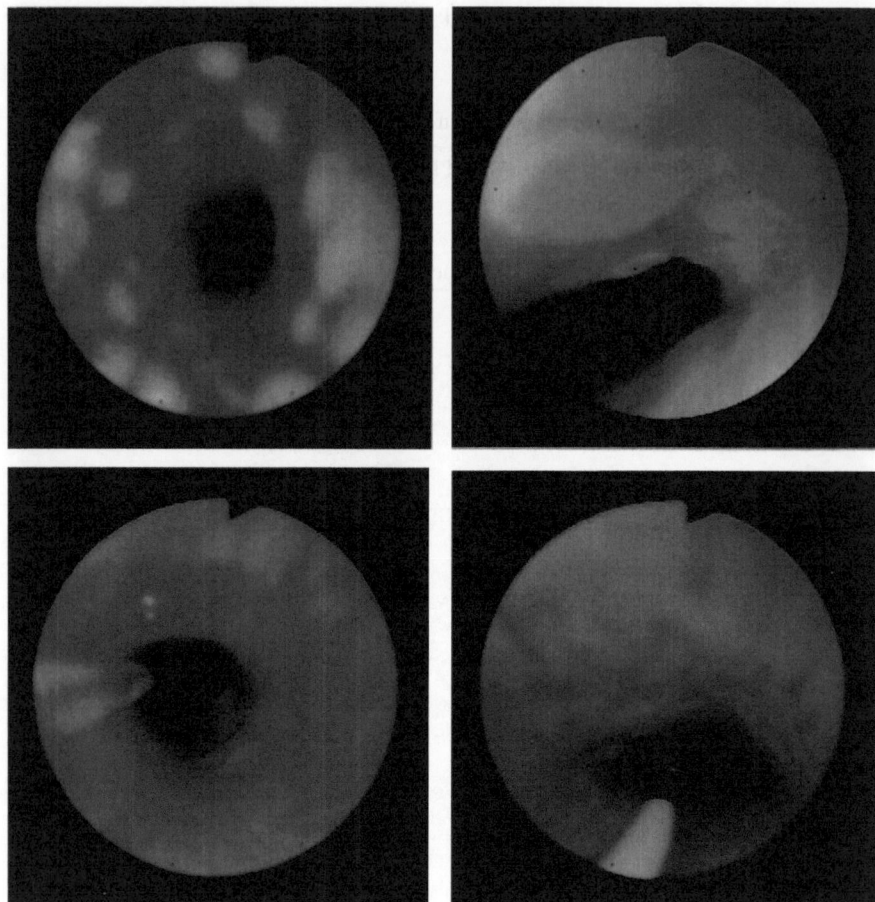

Fig. 4.1 (*upper left*). Flat, speckled, light depositions; early stage of atherosclerosis. No substantial stenosis. Only slightly irregular cross-section

Fig. 4.2 (*upper right*). Flat atherosclerotic plaques. The lumen of the vessel has lost its round shape but is not stenosed

Fig. 4.3 (*lower left*). Early atherosclerosis with mural depositions

Fig. 4.4 (*lower right*). Beginning sclerosis of the vascular wall

▶

Fig. 4.5 (*upper left*). Severe atherosclerosis with plaques almost completely occluding the vessel

Fig. 4.6 (*upper right*). Multiple atherosclerotic plaques without substantial vascular stenosis. Thrombotic deposition

Fig. 4.7 (*middle left*). Complicated atherosclerotic lesion with high-grade stenosis

Fig. 4.8 (*middle right*). Bedlike extension of plaques with flat or lumpy appearance

Fig. 4.9 (*lower left*). Flat circumscribed plaque with irregular vascular lumen

Fig. 4.10 (*lower right*). Eccentric stenosis with atherosclerotic plaque

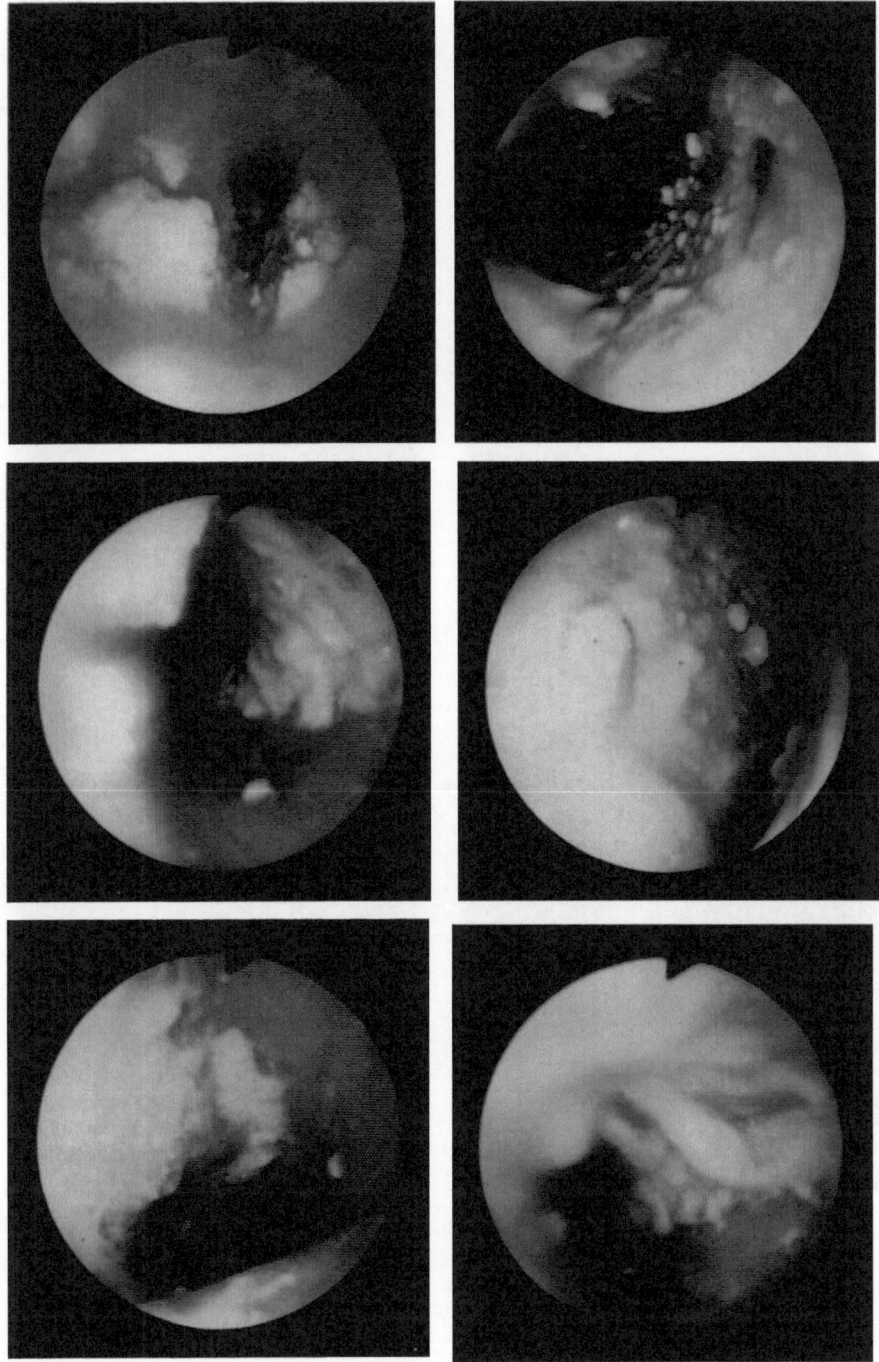

Figs. 4.5 to 4.10

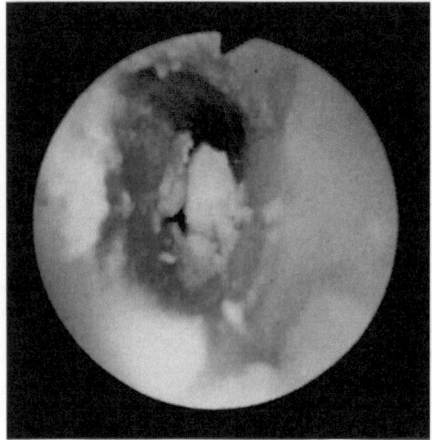

Fig. 4.11. An 85-year-old patient with arterial occlusive disease stage IV. Severe atherosclerotic plaques with almost complete occlusion of the vascular lumen

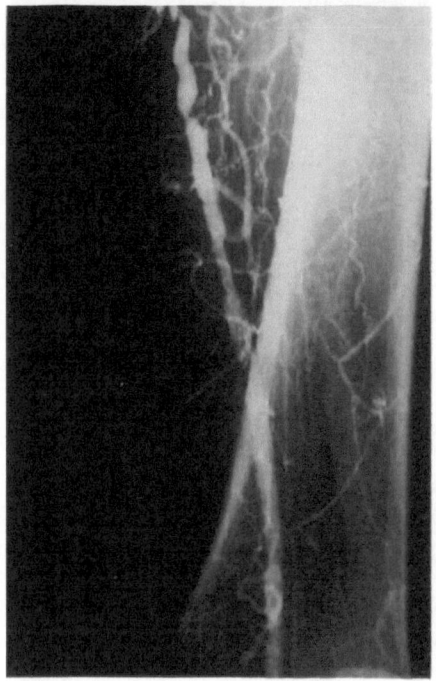

Fig. 4.12. Angiogram of the same patient as in Fig. 4.11. Atherosclerosis with high-grade stenosis of the superficial femoral artery

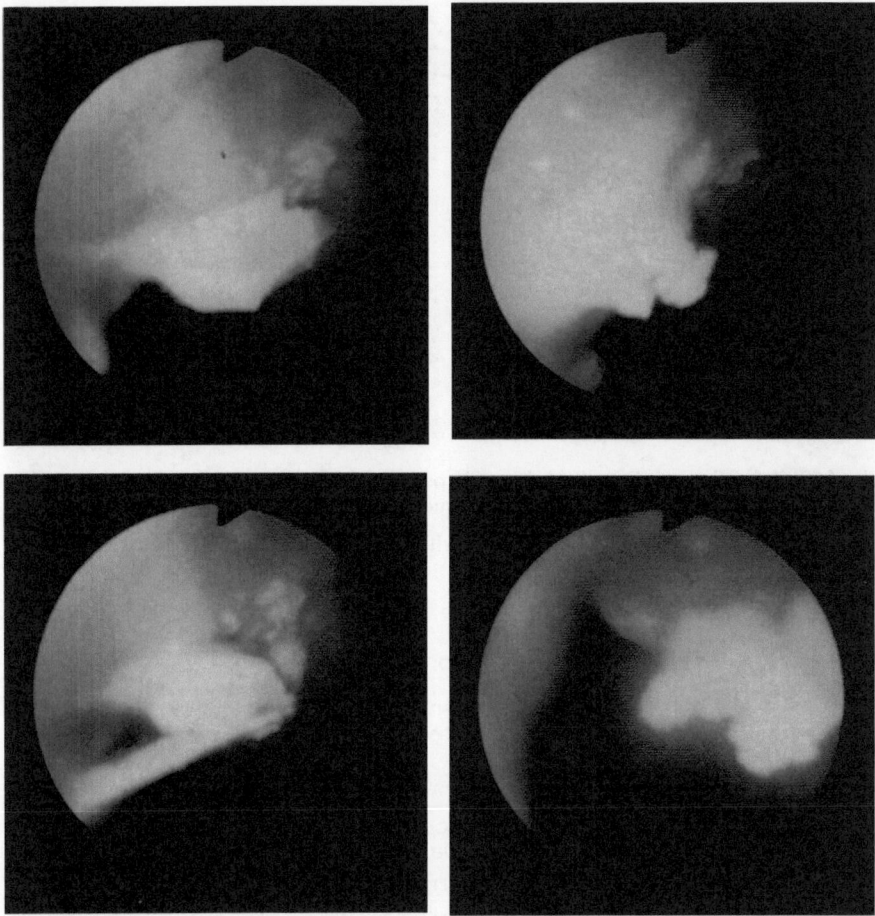

Fig. 4.13 (*upper left*). Eccentric plaques with broad basis

Fig. 4.14 (*upper right*). Two peaked atherosclerotic plaques shaped like stalactites

Fig. 4.15 (*lower left*). Angioscopic probing of a vessel. The wire cuts into the surface of the plaque

Fig. 4.16 (*lower right*). After removal of the wire the plaque is markedly notched

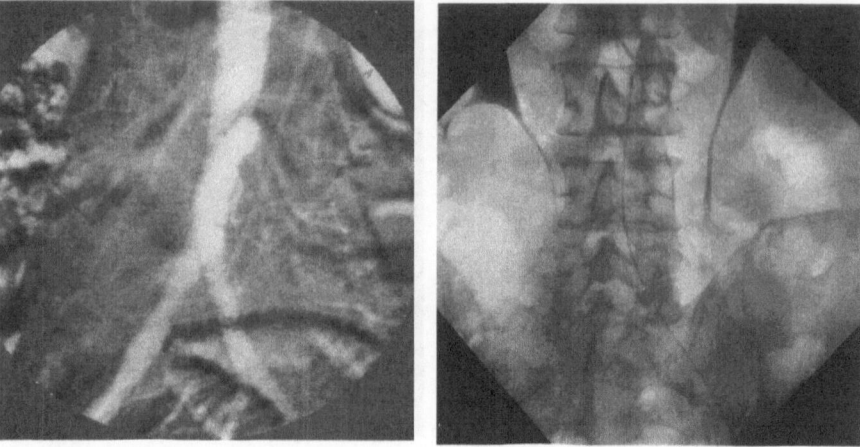

Fig. 4.17 (*left*). Severe ulcerative atherosclerosis of the abdominal aorta. Approximately 70% –80% stenosis caused by eccentric plaques

Fig. 4.18 (*right*). The endoscope is placed with its tip distally to the plaque. The blood flows primarily along the right side

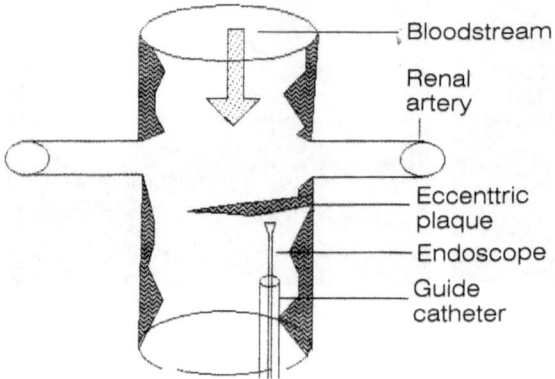

Fig. 4.19. Illustration of angioscopy of the aorta (bloodstream, renal artery, eccentric plaque, tip of the angioscope, guide catheter). Angioscopy in this special case was only possible because of a proximal eccentric plaque which reduced the blood flow so that a relatively small amount of sodium chloride flush of 20 ml was sufficient to clear the vascular lumen. Consequently, visualization of the aorta, the stenosis, and the plaque was only possible for a very short period between systole and diastole

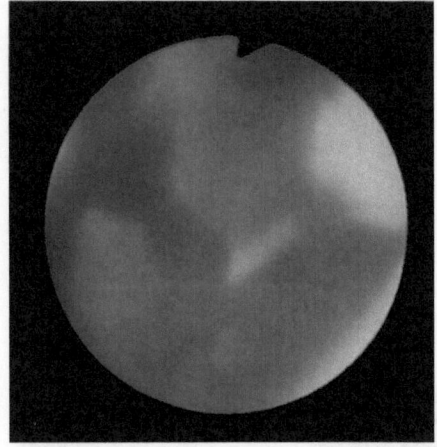

Fig. 4.20. Angioscopic image of a high-grade stenosis of the aorta caused by an atherosclerotic plaque

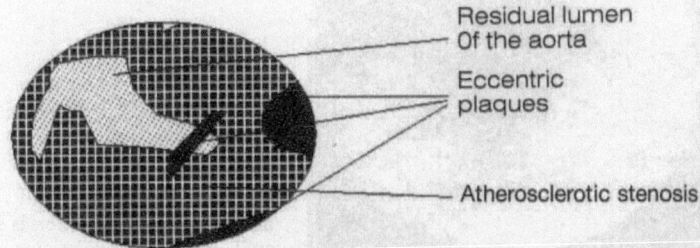

Residual lumen
Of the aorta

Eccentric
plaques

Atherosclerotic stenosis

Fig. 4.21. Diagram of the angioscopic image in Fig. 4.20

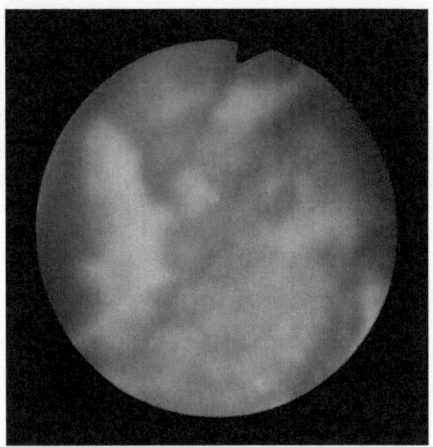

Fig. 4.22. Angioscopic illustration of an eccentric plaque

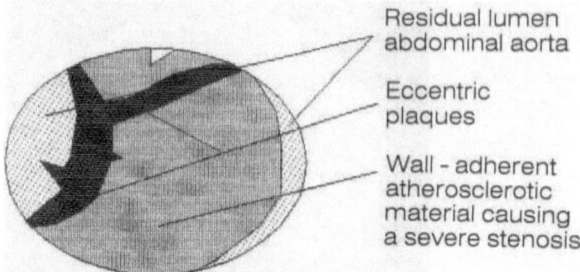

Residual lumen
abdominal aorta

Eccentric
plaques

Wall - adherent
atherosclerotic
material causing
a severe stenosis

Fig. 4.23. Diagram of
the angioscopic image
of Fig. 4.22

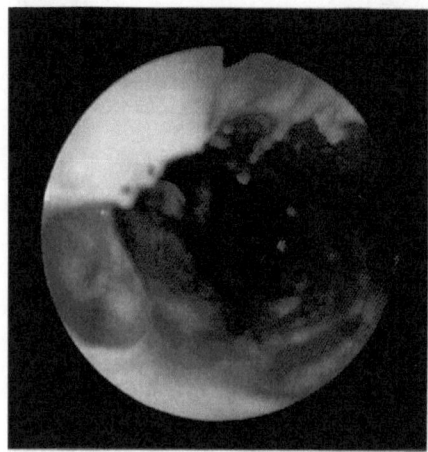

Fig. 4.24. Angioscopy of the residual
aortic lumen. The lumen is seen during a
split second between two systoles with
additional strong sodium chloride flush

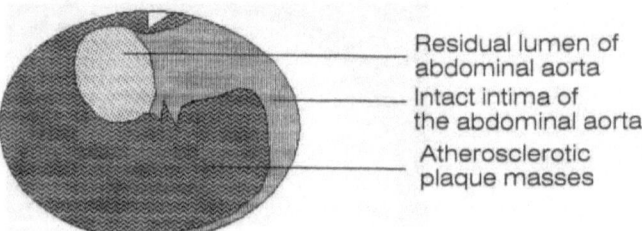

Residual lumen of
abdominal aorta

Intact intima of
the abdominal aorta

Atherosclerotic
plaque masses

Fig. 4.25. Diagram of the angioscopic image in Fig. 4.24

Fig. 4.27. Angioscopy with the characteristic feature of blurry angioscopic imaging caused
by floating and mural fibrin components

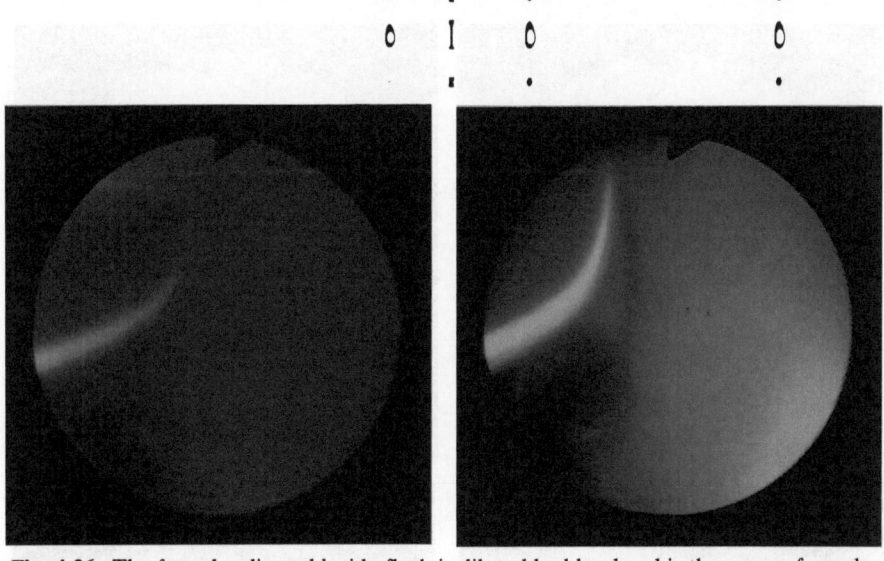

Fig. 4.26. The forced sodium chloride flush is diluted by blood and is the reason for only short-term view of mural thrombi

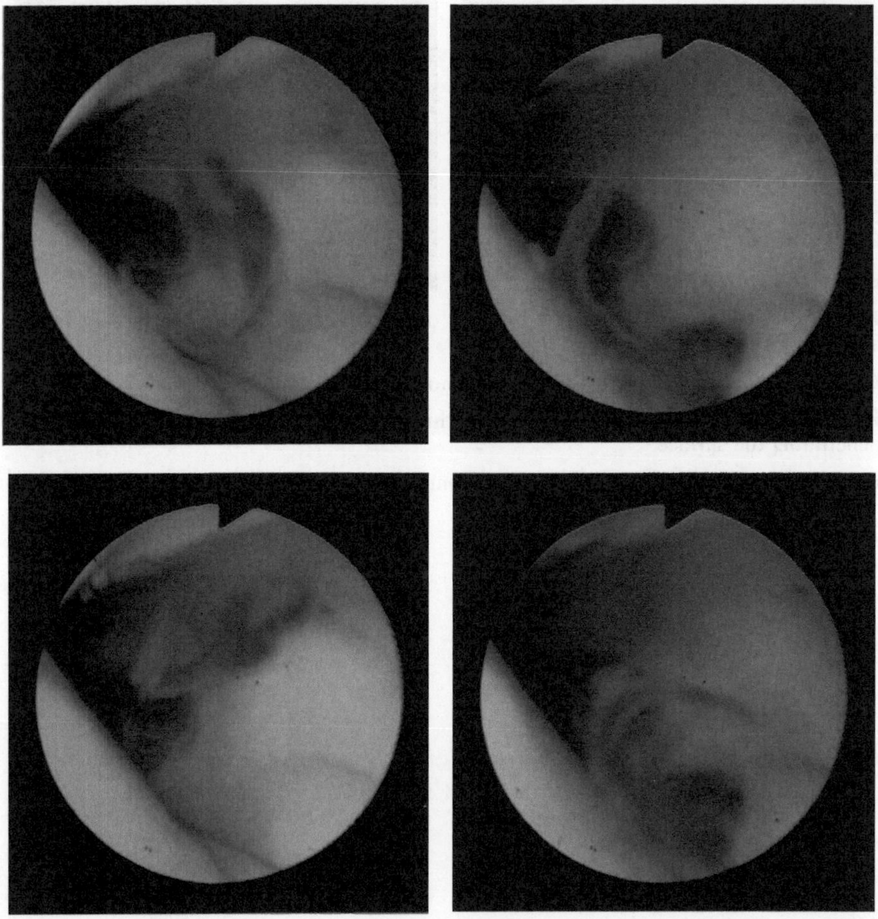

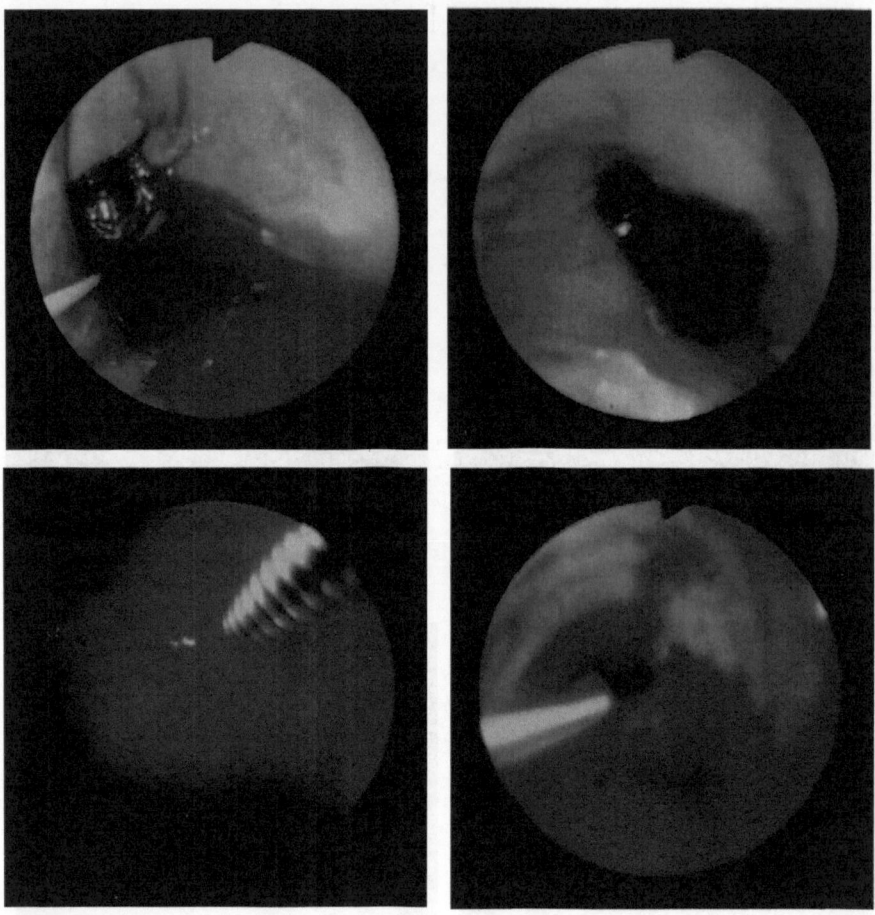

Fig. 4.28 (*upper left*). Angioscopic findings of a local thrombosis with fresh material adherent to the vascular wall

Fig. 4.29 (*upper right*). Occlusion of the femoral artery by an embolus

Fig. 4.30 (*lower left*). Fresh intravascular thrombotic material, the angioscopic wire penetrating the surface

Fig. 4.31 (*lower right*). Fresh adherent thrombus severely stenosing the vascular lumen

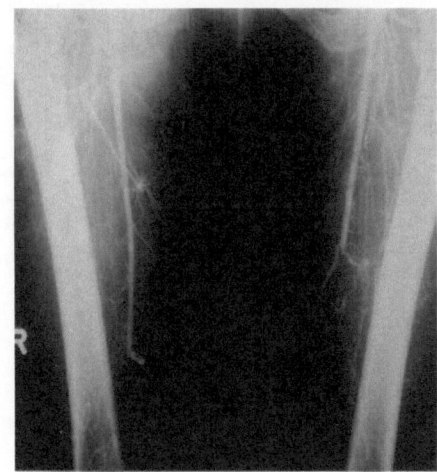

Fig. 4.32. Angiography of an 18-year-old women with thromboangiitis obliterans and arterial occlusive disease stage IV

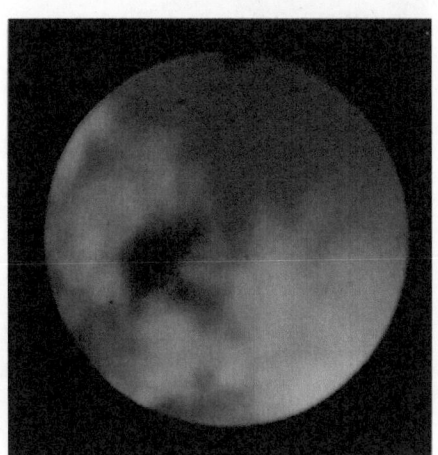

Fig. 4.33. Angioscopy of the same patient as in Fig. 4.32. High-grade stenosis of the femoral artery by cordlike and scarred intima

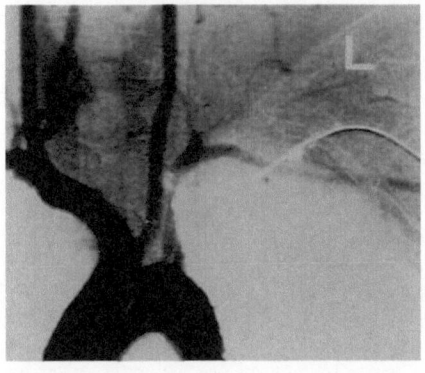

Fig. 4.34. A 64-year-old woman after radiotherapy of breast cancer. Arterial occlusive disease of the left arm with angiographically confirmed stenosis of the subclavian artery

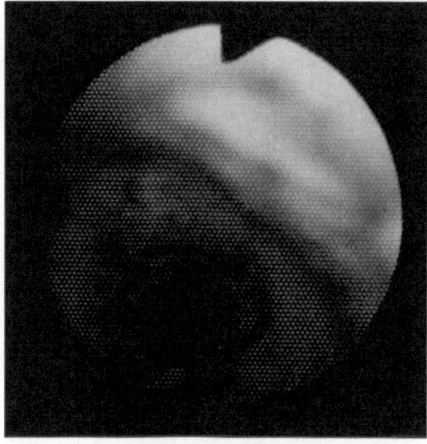

Fig. 4.35. Angioscopic finding of the same patient as in Fig. 4.34, with high-grade, long, and scarred stenosis

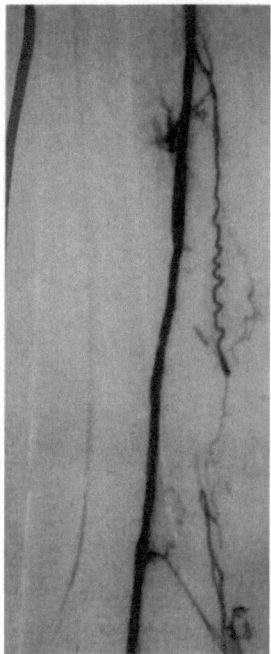

Fig. 4.36. Angiogram of a 54-year-old man with a myosarcoma of the thigh. The region had been treated with radiotherapy with 60 Gy. Multiple short stenoses of the femoral artery

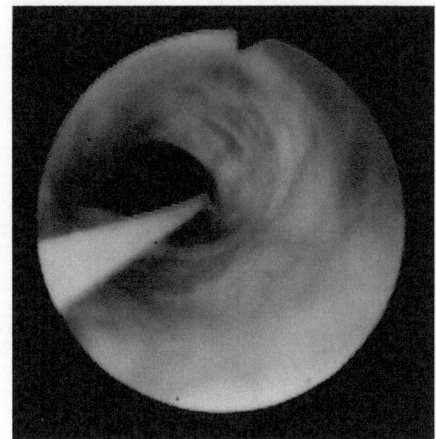

Fig. 4.37. Angioscopy of the same patient as in Fig. 4.36, showing scarred short stenoses with extensive disseminated scarring

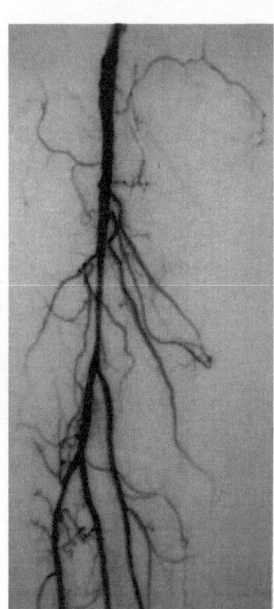

Fig. 4.38. A 50-year-old man suffering from a perosseous sarcoma. Angiographic finding after radiation therapy with 60 Gy. Angiography shows a long popliteal stenosis combined with an ectasia of the distal femoral artery

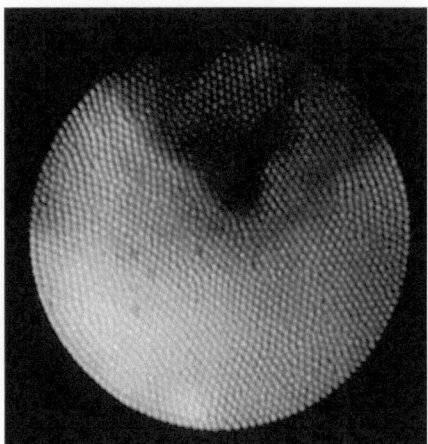

Fig. 4.39. Eccentric stenosis with an irregular rigid surface. At 3 o'clock a thrombotic lesion causes an eccentric stenosis narrowing the lumen more than 50%

5 Interventional Procedure in Angioscopy

Since Dotter and Judkins first introduced vascular dilatation, numerous attempts have been made to perform angioplasty in vivo and in vitro. Macroscopic as well as microscopic control could be performed only on postmortem tissue as PTA had not been employed. This problem was overcome by reducing the size of angioscopes to catheter sizes, and direct-control PTA by angioscopy became possible.

Furthermore, it had been desirable and necessary in many cases to achieve a direct vision of the dilated area to prevent imminent complications of PTA or local thrombolysis (Fig. 5.25a–c). Frequently, intravascular angiographic guide wire and catheter manipulations are performed. During such procedures complications, such as vascular dissections, are more easily recognized by angioscopy. Local thrombosis cannot be adequately distinguished from thromboembolism by angiography. Angioscopy is able to add substantial information and additionally enables lysis or extraction of the thrombus directly through the biopsy channel of the angioscope. Finally, the introduction of vascular stents has opened a new field for PTA as the procedure of implantation and especially the subsequent evaluation can be controlled by angioscopy.

5.1 The Method of PTA Control

Grüntzig's hypothesis that during balloon dilatation atheromatous plaques are compressed (as steps in fresh snow), changing the aggregate state of the plaque, has been refuted by histological analysis. Instead, balloon dilatation induces a dissection not only of the intima but also of the media. The cross-section of the vascular lumen thereby increases because of an increment in the entire vascular structure and the atheromatous plaques largely maintaining their configuration.

The results of PTA have been followed up by angioscopy in 41 patients. All of these had stage IIb–III (Fontaine) occlusive disease, and their vascular status had been morphologically documented by angiography. Atherosclerosis was the cause of vascular occlusions in 34 patients, four individuals had stenoses caused by radiotherapy of tumors, and three young patients had thromboangiitis obliterans. PTA was performed in the usual way with 5-F balloon catheters using the Seldinger technique, with the exception of using a femoral 8-F introducer sheath in all patients to facilitate the use of catheters and endoscopes. A precondition for safe angioscopy of higher grade stenoses or occlusions is introduction of the endoscope by the Seldinger technique. Replacing the angioscope by diagnostic and therapeutic catheters may in exceptional cases be carried out over a guide wire. The angioscope is handled exactly like a catheter. Changing the guide wire can be performed through the biopsy channel without difficulty. The relatively large tip of the angioscope, which does not taper off like a balloon catheter, cannot be advanced to the higher grade stenoses without a guide wire because of the risk of dissection or vascular occlusion. Another precondition for angioscopy of a vessel stenosis is X-ray control. If resistance is noticed on advancing the endoscope that cannot be overcome even under radiological control with contrast medium, the procedure must be discontinued and a conventional PTA undertaken before another attempt with angioscopy can be made.

Of 119 dilatations, 132 were performed in the femoral and popliteal region. The technical conditions were markedly better in the antegrade than in the retrograde puncture direction of the pelvic area. In the retrograde technique a balloon catheter had first to be placed above the puncture site in crossover technique from the contralateral femoral artery to block the proximal blood flow before angioscopy could be performed from the ipsilateral side (Fig. 3.5). The endoscope was advanced through the introducer sheath before and after the dilatation and the vascular lumen visualized after an angioscopic sodium chloride flush. Furthermore, in five cases when it was impossible to place the guide wire into the distal vessel, the wire was directed through the biopsy channel of the endoscope to that site under direct angioscopic view. In the supra-aortic regions (Fig. 3.4) a 9-F guiding catheter with a large lumen had to be positioned before the endoscope was advanced through the catheter (Fig. 5.1).

In one patient angioscopy was used to facilitate insertion of a guide wire into a renal artery which could not be entered safely by angiography. The technical procedure was comparable to that of supra-aortic vessels. Through a 9-F introducer sheath an 8-F catheter was selectively placed directly in front of the renal artery. Radiographs were first taken of the renal artery before the angioscope was advanced through the catheter to the proximal renal artery

Table 5.1. Summary of angioscopic vascular results after PTA

Minor ability to compress atheroma
Extension of the vascular lumen by tearing
Atherosclerotic plaques (primarily longitudinal, rarely circular tears)
Increased instability of the vascular wall when the lumen has a slitlike cross-section
Wall-adherent thrombi in tears of atheromatous plaques that have been caused by PTA
Possible embolization of prominent atherosclerotic plaques
Possible embolization of wall-adherent thrombi
Increment of blood flow after successful dilatation
Inflammatory and actinic vascular stenoses not as successfully dilated as stenoses of other origin because of extensive scarring

(Figs. 5.2, 5.3). Because of the large diameter of the catheter the blood flow within the renal artery is almost completely stopped so that a sodium chloride flush of 15 ml through the biopsy channel is only needed to achieve a visualization time of 3–5 s. This is sufficient to allow the guide wire to be positioned precisely in the renal artery. After dilatation of the stenosis the balloon catheter was replaced by the angioscope using the Seldinger technique and leaving the guide wire in place. The result was visualized by angioscopy (Figs. 5.2–5.3).

5.2 Angioscopic Results After PTA

Angioscopy performed after dilation of vascular stenoses has revealed several results which had not been diagnosed unequivocally before.

1. Atheromatous plaques can be compressed only partly by balloon dilatation. Peaked atheromas are easier to change in their configuration than flat plaques. Merely probing with wires can notch prominent atheromatous plaques (Figs. 5.10–5.13).
2. After dilatation of atherosclerotic plaques, angioscopy enables evaluation of different types of tears of varying severity (Figs. 5.4–5.19). Tears are longitudinal in about 90% and circular in about 20% of cases (Fig. 5.11). The longitudinal fissures depend on the length of the balloon (Figs. 5.7a, 5.15, 5.19).
3. Long tears running through atheromatous plaques cause vascular instability after dilatation. Vascular stenoses can generally be extended by dilatation even though eccentric stenoses are sometimes left (Figs. 5.11–5.14). On compression from the outside the lumen seems markedly more unstable than prior to the dilatation. If several stenoses are dilated, this phenomenon is even more striking as that part with the most tearings has the least stability. Dilatation of the vascular lumen above its original size impairs the general vascular situation by reducing the stability of the atherosclerotic vessel. Despite good positioning of the catheter and successful dilatation an immediately recurrent stenosis or occlusion can be explained by this mechanism.
4. Thrombotic material adherent to the vessel wall is often found within tears of atherosclerotic plaques after dilatation. The detachment with sodium chloride flush is markedly delayed. These thrombi are present especially in the stenosing area and are responsible for early restenosing as well as thrombotic occlusion of the vascular lumen.
5. During dilatation of prominent atherosclerotic plaques parts of these plaques can break off and cause peripheral embolism. This can be seen on simple probing with a guide wire (Figs. 5.10, 5.11). Long atherosclerotic stenoses exceeding 2 cm with eccentric plaques are prone to this complication (Figs. 5.20–5.24).
6. Parts of the thrombus can break off during balloon dilatation and can cause peripheral embolism. This phenomenon must be suspected when mural thrombi seen prior to PTA are absent after the procedure.

7. Even though dilatation of a long stenosis expands the vascular lumen, the vascular surface becomes ragged after PTA (Fig. 5.24). This is the cause of prolonged adherence of blood components seen at angioscopy after PTA.
8. Angioscopic control shows an increase in blood flow after PTA. This is reflected by an increase in sodium chloride flush required.
9. Dilatations of actinic vascular changes are only partly successful as the vascular regions stenosed by scarring are still relatively elastic so that the extension of the cross-section by PTA is only short-lived and quickly returns to the starting point (Table 5.1).

5.3 Method for Lysis Control

Since 1982, 440 angiographically controlled local lysis procedures have been performed at Freiburg University Hospital. In the past 4 years, local lysis of the lower extremity with additional angioscopic control was carried out in 30 animal studies and in 43 patients. For this purpose several ultrathin angioscopes have been available with outside diameters of 1.5–2.2 mm and a biopsy channel with diameters of 0.35–0.5 mm. Through the biopsy channels of the angioscopes thin guide wires can be inserted, and thrombolytic agents such as urokinase or streptokinase can be directly infused. The results of the lysis are evaluated every hour by angioscopy and by angiography. Invariably we use the procedure of percutaneous puncture of the femoral artery rather than earlier methods in which the vessels must be opened surgically.

The aim of this study was, first, to achieve a method combining percutaneous angiography, angioscopy, and lysis therapy without exposing the patient to more than a routine catheter lysis. A second aim was to distinguish thromboembolism from local thrombosis by angioscopy. This is often impossible by angiography alone. Our third aim was to determine whether angioscopy is capable of visualizing the vascular status after local lysis or after possible subsequent vascular dilatation.

After puncture of the femoral artery and subsequent introduction of a 7- to 8-F introducer sheath in an antegrade direction, a straight 5-F lysis catheter was advanced over a guide wire in the Seldinger technique to the thrombus. The lysis catheter was then replaced by an angioscope, leaving the guide wire in place. Physiological sodium chloride solution with a constantly monitored pressure of 300 mmHg was injected through the biopsy channel of the angioscope for good visualization. Afterwards the guide wire was advanced through the thrombus under angioscopic and radiological control. Local lysis was performed with a dose of 25 000 U streptokinase or 100 000 U urokinase per hour with hourly monitoring of fibrinogen levels and thrombin and reptilase times. Urokinase or streptokinase were perfused through the biopsy channel of the angioscope by a perfusion pump. The tip of the angioscope was positioned 2 cm proximal to the thrombus. The result was evaluated every hour by angioscopy and by angiography.

Prior to the use in patients this method of local lysis through the biopsy channel of an angioscope had been evaluated in 30 animal studies. Because of the diminished vision during angioscopy of vascular thrombotic occlusions caused by thrombotic particles whirled up by the angioscopic flushing sodium chloride this method had to be evaluated before its use in patients. In animal studies local thrombosis was induced by injecting a local thrombotic agent (2% Ethoxysclerol) into the iliac artery, which had been occluded by a balloon catheter for 5 min. Additional manual compression caused a local vascular thrombosis to be induced. In animals a complete thrombotic occlusion of the iliac artery was achieved in this manner. After advancing the angioscope through the femoral introducer sheath into the femoral artery the local thrombosis was visualized. With a constant sodium chloride infusion and additional intravascular injection of 200 000 U streptokinase over 30 min the thrombosis could be completely opened under direct angioscopic view.

The successful local lysis performed through an angioscope can be recorded on videotape. Peripheral embolization of thrombus particles can be demonstrated. This information cannot be obtained by angiography, and embolization can be proven only by arterial occlusion of the periphery.

5.4 Angioscopic Results of Local Lysis

None of the 43 patients who underwent local catheter lysis via an angioscope suffered complications. The output and quality of the angioscopic photographs and tapes were variable. All angioscopic photographs were taken using a sodium chloride flush so that the quality was not comparable to those of gastroscopy where visualization is optimized by air insufflation. In particular the visualization of intravascular thrombi is limited as particles of the thrombotic surface are constantly detached throughout the procedure. In contrast, angioscopy of a patent vessel is far better as the blood sodium chloride solution runs off in seconds and gives good view of the vessel (Figs. 5.26–5.36).

A striking finding was that the surface of the vascular thrombi was relatively firm and shiny (Figs. 5.28–5.29). Injection of sodium chloride solution did not markedly change the surface features. Initial perforation of the thrombus with the guide wire is essential and a precondition for successful lysis since in this situation the fibrinolytic agents have been shown to be more effective (Fig. 5.31). This finding underlines the fact that local lysis should be initiated directly at the thrombus as fibrinolytic agents otherwise escape through collateral vessels. A local thrombosis which has developed as the result of a high-grade atherosclerotic stenosis in combination with reduced blood flow or stasis can be differentiated from an embolus by angioscopy. An appositional mural thrombus has a characteristic appearance: conglomerates of platelets form a coral-like lamellar network covered and entangled by fibrin layers like a "bracing architecture." The platelet conglomerates project over the surface of the thrombus, appearing like a corrugation crosswise to the direction of the bloodstream (sandbank relief). The color is mostly grayish red (Figs. 5.28–5.31, 5.35). The coagulation thrombus is generally red to black on angioscopy and shows a regular, wall-adherent structure with a homogeneous surface. An embolus, on the other hand, has an inhomogeneous surface, lacks characteristic color, and differs in its lysis characteristics (Figs. 5.32–5.34).

A continuously developing appositional thrombus can be dissolved from the proximal to the distal end whereas a prominent embolus with an irregular consistency can be dissolved only protractedly or not at all.

Comparing angiography and angioscopy in the control local lysis angioscopy reveals serious pathological changes of the arterial wall, especially when dilatation is performed in addition to previous lysis. Ulceration of the intima, residual plaques, and fibrinoid apposition favor the adherence of platelets and the development of recurrent thrombus occlusion or stenosis. In cases of severe pathological vascular changes, especially in the region of the femoral and popliteal arteries, application of an additional vascular endoprosthesis is sensible especially when the residual stenosis can be dilated only inadequately by balloon catheterization, the irregular lumen measures only 2–3 mm, or mural thrombotic material can be removed only partly or not at all.

In arterial thrombolysis angioscopy has proven not to add to complications. The rule of thumb is that an angioscope can be placed without additional harm in a vessel in which a catheter can be placed (Table 5.2).

Table 5.2. Comparison of angioscopy and angiography in local catheter thrombolysis

	Angioscopy	Angiography
Dosage of fibrinolytic agents	+	+
Perforation of the thrombus by a guide wire	+	+
Permanent control of lysis,	+	(+)
therapeutic success seen immediately	+	+
Diagnosis of residual thrombosis	+	(+)
Diagnosis of cause of stenosis:		
atherosclerosis, inflammation, actinic injury	+	(+)
Assessment of the outflow tract after local lysis	−	+
Diagnosis of peripheral embolization after thrombolysis	(+)	+
Reduction of contrast medium	(+)	−
Reduction of radiation	(+)	−

+, Certain advantage; (+), possible advantage; −, disadvantage

5.5 Method of Stent Implantation

An innovation in the therapy of arterial occlusive disease are intraluminal expandable vascular prostheses. These devices have been constructed to help prevent early recurrent occlusion after angioplasty that is caused by the elastic vascular structure, progressive intimal proliferation, and excessive vascular scarring. Three basic types of stents have been developed:

1. One stent model is made from a steel lattice with plastic deformability. The stent is expanded by inflation of a balloon catheter and fixed within the stenosed vascular area. Because of the stent's highly elastic structure, elastic recoiling of the dilated vessel is prevented.
2. The second type of stent is designed to keep a dilated stenosis open, based on the principle of elastic self-expansion after withdrawing the catheter. The stent is made from a thermolabile metal that is introduced into the vessel in frozen condition and expands to its original size at 37°C blood temperature ("memory metal").
3. The elasticity of the above stents is maintained after intravascular implantation, so that recurrent stenosis of the vascular lumen cannot always be prevented; especially when applied to firm atherosclerotic stenoses or occlusions the stents can easily collapse. For this reason a third type of stent was developed at Freiburg University Hospital which is also based on the principle of plastic deformability by a special balloon catheter, but which differs in material, mechanism of expansion, and stability from the previous models.

Recurrent stenoses and occlusions after PTA often vary in location and severity depending on the vascular region. In particular in the distal parts of the superficial femoral and popliteal artery long-term results have been shown to be worse than in central vascular regions. Frequently an unfavorable prognosis can be predicted directly after PTA, especially when severe, long and high-grade stenoses remain after the procedure. The prognosis can be improved only by achieving a relatively stable and long-lasting vascular dilatation. The current types of endoprostheses still reveal important weak points regarding stability so that more durable stents had to be developed. This innovation has been promoted by the Department of Diagnostic Radiology of Freiburg University Hospital over the past 3 years. Numerous problems had to be solved during this time regarding material; deformability, stability, and transfemoral application of the stents. Major problems have been the recurrent thrombosis or stenosis of the endoprosthetic lumen. These difficulties first had to be overcome in animal experiments.

The basic materials for the vascular stents are brass and silver. These are formed to a framework 0.2 mm thick which is compressed to 0.14 mm; the edges are silver-bordered to prevent fraying out of the stent within the vessel. The stent is designed to be expanded longitudinally with the frame wires in a parallel position. Oblique or rhombic structure of the lattice is disadvantageous on expansion of the stents and must be avoided. Additionally, two cross-pieces are soldered with silver into the brass lattice. All edges are rounded off under a phase microscope and soldered again if necessary. After successive mechanical compression the stent has a thickness of less than 0.14 mm (Fig. 5.37). The lattice must be severely compressed to smooth out the rough surface for smooth mechanical expansion of the stent by a balloon dilatation (Figs. 5.38, 5.39). The plane lattice is then wrapped around a deflated balloon of a 5-F/7-F Olbert catheter. The length of the prosthesis equals that of the balloon. Then the stability of the prosthesis-catheter construction is inspected manually and checked for smooth crossing through an 8-F introducer sheath (Figs. 5.40, 5.41). Later the endoprosthesis is placed via the transfemoral route into the vessel. After puncture of the femoral artery an 8-F introducer sheath is placed within the vessel, and a guide wire is advanced across the stenosed segment of the vessel. The balloon catheter with the stent is advanced to the stenosis, and the lesion is dilated with a pressure of 6 bar under radiological control. After dilatation the stent is firmly anchored in the stenosed region by its own elastic tension.

5.6 Angioscopic Results of Stent Implantation

5.6.1 Angioscopic Stent Implantation and Control in Animal Experiments

Our vascular endoprostheses have been introduced into 18 vascular regions of four dogs. The stents were advanced into the arteries by transfemoral route through 8-F introducer sheaths with the assistance of 7-F (4 cm/12 mm) balloon catheters. In each dog five stents were implanted into the iliac artery, femoral artery, abdominal aorta, vena cava, and carotid artery. The stents measured 4–13 mm in intraluminal diameter and were positioned under radiological control over an 8-F introducer sheath. All stents could be introduced transfemorally without difficulty to the desired site by angioscopy. The results of stent implantation were examined every 2–3 months by angiography and by angioscopy. Questions concerning new intima development, restenosing, and thrombosis, often difficult to evaluate by angiography, have been answered by angioscopy.

Immediately after implanting the stents good pulses were felt in distal arteries. Transfemoral angioscopic examination was performed after 2 days and 4 weeks with ultrathin endoscopes, 1.9 mm in diameter. To undertake this procedure a special technique for emptying the vessel of blood was developed to achieve a short angioscopic view of the vessel. Follow-up examinations revealed patent stents in all cases after 2 days and after 4 weeks. However, in three cases the stents were partially restenosed by thrombosis. After 4 weeks a new intimal lining covered part of the lattice, but the remaining portion looked metallic. Occasionally thrombotic depositions, 1 mm in diameter, were seen in small recesses of the stent lattice, but they did not stenose the vascular lumen. There was no intima reaction, stenosis, or thrombosis at the site of the original vascular wall or edge of the stent. Neither ulceration of the intima caused by local injury at the edge of the stent nor distal dislocation of the stent were observed. During the angioscopic examination the stent was cautiously touched with the tip of the angioscope. In none of the cases was loosening or dislocation of the stent evident. Histological examination was not performed since all animals are still alive. Follow-up is now over 8 months (Fig. 5.42).

5.6.2 Angioscopic Stent Implantation and Control in Patients

Angioscopy was performed during stent implantation and during long-term examinations. Stent follow-up examinations should be performed expediently by angiography and angioscopy as the blood flow and positioning of the stent can easily be controlled by angiography whereas restenosis or thrombosis can be evaluated best by angiography. In all, four patients were treated with the new type of stent in the Consiglio Nazionale delle Richerche in Rome together with Dr. Milic. Four patients were examined by angiography and three by angioscopy (Figs. 5.43–5.45). The vascular stenoses were located in the inguinal region (two), the femoral region (one), and the distal popliteal artery (one). In all these patients recurrent dilatations in these vascular regions had been attempted unsuccessfully. After extensive review and discussion of acute und chronic complications of intravascular stent implantation with the patient and pointing out the alternative of surgical revision the stent implantation was carried out. At follow-up examination it was important to determine stent position and patency, the degree of stenosis or thrombosis, and intimal formation within the stent.

For stent implantation into the superficial femoral artery and the popliteal artery (Figs. 5.47–5.53) the femoral artery was punctured above and below the inguinal ligament, and a 7-F introducer sheath with the angioscope and an 8-F introducer sheath with the stent on a balloon catheter were introduced. The insertion of stents into the iliac arteries was conducted only under angiographic and radiological control, while the control examinations of stent implantation were performed by angioscopy in the manner described above.

Angioscopic long-term follow-up studies were undertaken after 3 months; initial intimal formation covering the metal lattice (Fig. 5.53) could be seen. Final results about this type of therapy are not yet sufficient because control studies have only been under way for 8 months. Further long-term results of stent implantation are necessary for definitive assessment of the benefits of this procedure.

On examination up to 40% of the metal stent structure was covered by a grayish-white layer with partial adhesion of small thrombotic particles (Figs. 5.52). Features of atherosclerosis and thrombosis were seen within the stents. Other parts of the stent maintained their metallic appearance. The vascular wall adjacent to the stent had a normal appearance and showed no sign of ulceration. Control examination of the stents confirmed that a free run-off of the angioscopic flush unequivocally indicates a good function of the stent. The longest follow-up of successful stent implantation in humans into the distal popliteal artery and the femoral artery is currently 20 months. The clinical symptoms of these two patients were markedly improved. In the iliac region the longest follow-up interval is 24 months, also with good clinical results (Table 5.3).

Table 5.3. Summary of the angioscopic findings of the intravascular stent control. (Stent by Beck and Nanko, Freiburg University Hospital, FRG)

Immediate control (during stent implantation)
   Procedure of stent implantation
   Control of position of stent
   Control of intravascular fastening
   Control of blood flow after stent implantation

Late control (at earliest after 3 months)
   Assessment of new intimal layer
   Assessment of recurring stenosis
   Assessment of thrombosis
   Control of adjacent vessel
   Control of position of stent
   Assessment of blood flow

5.7 The Invention of a Method of Percutaneous Transluminal Thrombus Extraction and Its Angioscopic Control

5.7.1 Principle, Material, and Method

Interventional radiology sometimes faces insoluble problems in the treatment of arterial thrombosis by local catheter lysis, such as the difficulty of transfemoral access, small catheters, limitation in thrombolytic doses, limited time for the procedure, old thrombotic lysis or thromboembolism, and dilatation of residual stenoses after local lysis. These problems may make local lysis impossible and demand a further therapeutic procedure.

For the past 2 years our research group at Freiburg University Hospital has been working on a mechanical device for breaking up intravascular thrombosis. This tool has been shown to remove large amounts of thrombotic material from an artery through a transfemoral catheter without an additional burden or risk for the patient. Later a local lysis with reduction in doses of urokinase or streptokinase can follow. This idea of breaking up large amounts of thrombotic material by mechanical means, subsequently extracting this material, and later initiating thrombolysis with a reduced dose developed because long thrombotic occlusions can be opened only with high doses of urokinase or streptokinase. By mechanical manipulation of the thrombus this dose can be reduced, and the risk of higher dose thrombolysis can be avoided. The aim was to design a drilling device which could be introduced through a catheter lumen to the thrombosis, and which would simultaneously break up and aspirate solid thrombotic material by vacuum suction without damaging the vascular wall. We succeeded in constructing such a device whose function has been tested in vitro and in vivo. In clinical cases this technique was controlled by angioscopy with concomitant angiography.

The thrombus extraction device operates within a straight 7.5-F catheter, 1 m in length. The tip of the catheter is open and has no distal tapering. A guide wire, 0.6 mm in diameter, is placed which has a tip consisting of a drilling device with five windings (Fig. 5.54). The guide wire inserted into the catheter has several soldered joints from the tip to the proximal end at 4 cm spacing to achieve a good and safe winding stability. The distal coil is 1.4 mm thick and 2 cm long and is plugged onto the guide wire and soldered several times so that rotation within the catheter is possible. Between the guide wire and the distal drilling device a space of 0.5 mm is left. This construction allows a smooth rotation of the drilling device. The tip of the guide wire never leaves the end of the catheter during the drilling so that a perforation of the vascular wall is prevented. The proximal part of the catheter has a double lumen, one for the guide wire and one for the suction equipment that produces a negative pressure within the catheter during the rotation procedure (Fig. 5.55). The guide wire is connected at the proximal end with a small electric motor with a variable speed of transmission from 15 to 20 000 RPM. This allows rotation of the wire inside the catheter almost without vibration. The electric motor measures only 5×2 cm and weighs 140 g. To achieve the safest and most comfortable handling the motor is soldered onto a metal pistol handle with a polyurethane surface so that the device can be handled with one hand (Fig. 5.56).

During thrombus extraction a variable rotational speed of 5 – 50 RPM is electronically set. A roller pump is connected to the second catheter exit for continuous suction. The coiling of the drilling device together with simultaneous suction allows aspiration and destruction of thrombotic material. This material is then removed by aspiration of the pump. This process is supported by the movement of the tip of the catheter by 2 – 3 mm which can be started by the pulling the trigger of the device. By this mechanism thrombus material is mechanically drawn into the catheter in addition to the vacuum aspiration (Figs. 5.57, 5.58). The in vitro experiments with two human apposition thrombi 3 cm in diameter show easy aspiration and subsequent intraluminal destruction of the thrombotic material to pieces of less than 0.5 mm (Fig. 5.59).

Preconditions for the use of this method are transfemoral access through an 8-F introducer sheath and precise positioning of the catheter tip into the thrombus under direct angioscopic view and X-ray control. Furthermore, detailed knowledge of the vascular system and the site and length of the thrombus is mandatory for thrombus extraction and must be recorded by arterial angiography. Reducing the size of the catheter made possible thrombus extraction under angioscopic view in animals. Reduction of the thrombus extraction catheters from 7-F to 5-F systems was technically difficult since the space between the coil and the catheter wall as well as the depth of the coil had to be reduced. Both factors are of major importance in the extraction of thrombotic material.

5.7.2 Angioscopic and Angiosgraphic Results in Animal Studies and Clinical Experience in Patients

Percutaneous extraction by aspiration of thrombotic material with subsequent local thrombolysis (Figs. 5.60–5.62) was performed successfully in animals as well as in 58 patients. The procedure is illustrated by angioscopy in animal studies. At first the visible thrombus is aspirated under angioscopic control and cut into pieces within the catheter until most of the thrombotic material is removed (Figs. 5.63–5.65). The coil is not visible during the entire process to prevent damage to the vascular wall. The thrombi of the patients were all located in the femoral and popliteal vascular system as far distally as the trifurcation and extended over a length from 2 mm to 9 cm. We achieved recanalization of the vascular lumen by aspiration extraction thrombectomy in all patients. In one patient almost 20 g of partly fresh and partly old thrombotic material was extracted. Complications such as dissection, perforation, or catheter-induced thrombosis were not observed in any patient. The results were controlled immediately by angioscopy. At 2- to 4-month follow-up a good clinical result was still present.

Because major parts of the thrombus were extracted, the doses of local thrombolysis, urokinase, or streptokinase could be reduced. In half of the cases the administration of local thrombolytic agents was not necessary in addition to thrombus extraction. When it was additionally needed, thrombolysis was performed with 250 000 U streptokinase and 750 000 U urokinase (in 50 % of the individuals). Both angioscopy and angiography confirmed the recanalization of the vascular lumen after the procedures. No vascular wall injury was observed (Figs. 5.66–5.71). Complications did not occur with this method. This was expected as there was no additional risk to the patient compared with routine catheter angiography, and the risk for the patient was further reduced by diminishing the dose of the local lysis medication.

5.8 Other Possibilities for the Use of Vascular Intraluminal Angioscopy

Endovascular control of the new interventional procedures such as the rotation devices for reopening occluded arteries has been shown to be a developing field for intraluminal endoscopy. In our hospital we are currently using two rotation systems, the ROTACS system with slow rotation speed and the Beck system with high rotation speed. In one patient with a long distal occlusion of the femoral and popliteal artery angiography revealed interesting results. After thrombus extraction by rotation angioplasty the vascular wall was severely injured, and endoluminal thrombotic adhesions were observed. The vascular injury appeared to be mainly circular, but longitudinal intimal fissures were also present. These observations show that previous opinions neglecting intravascular damage of arteries by interventional manipulation are obviously wrong (Figs. 5.72, 5.73; Table 5.4).

Table 5.4. Summary of possible indications for angioscopy in addition to percutaneous thrombus extraction

Direct control of thrombus extraction
Control of additional vascular changes atherosclerosis, inflammation, embolism
Evaluation of the residual thrombosis
Indication for additional local lysis
Indication for additional vascular dilatation
Possible long-term control
With reduction of the extraction catheter size (4–5 F), which is currently only possible in animals, thrombus extraction may eventually be controlled under direct angioscopic view

Endoluminal control of vascular surgical therapy was first reported by Vollmar [384] as an additional intraoperative method with excellent results. Especially in some patients postoperative endoluminal examination of vascular sutures in the anastomotic region may be very helpful (Figs. 5.74–5.100).

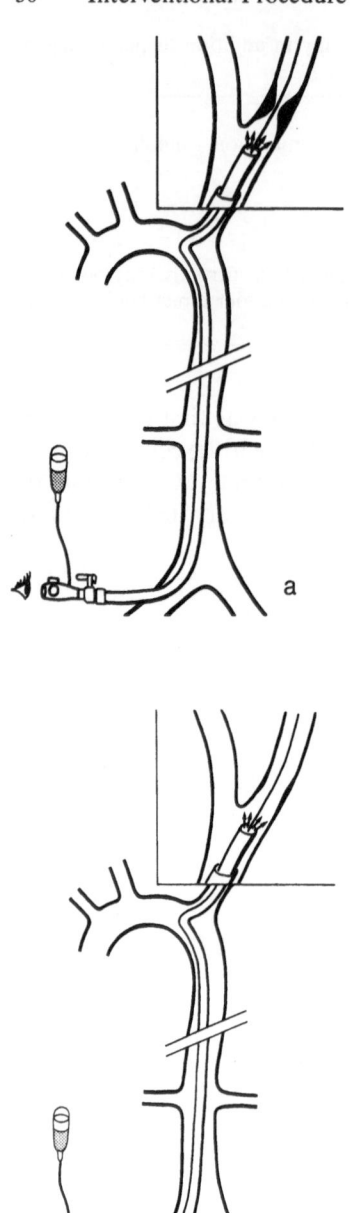
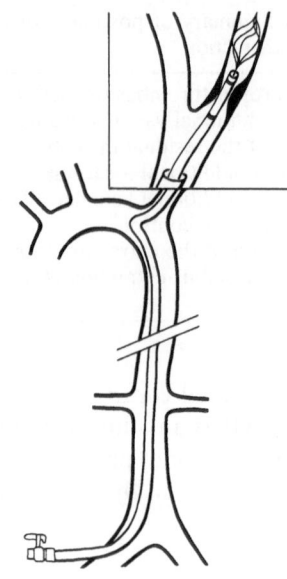

Fig. 5.1a–c. Technical procedure of dilatation and angioscopy of supra-aortic vessels. **a** The endoscope is advanced through an 8-F guide catheter to the region of interest. **b** Replacement of the endoscope by a dilatation catheter. Under the protection of a thrombic filter, developed by Nanko and Beck, the carotid artery is dilated. **c** Replacement of the catheter by an endoscope and angioscopic control

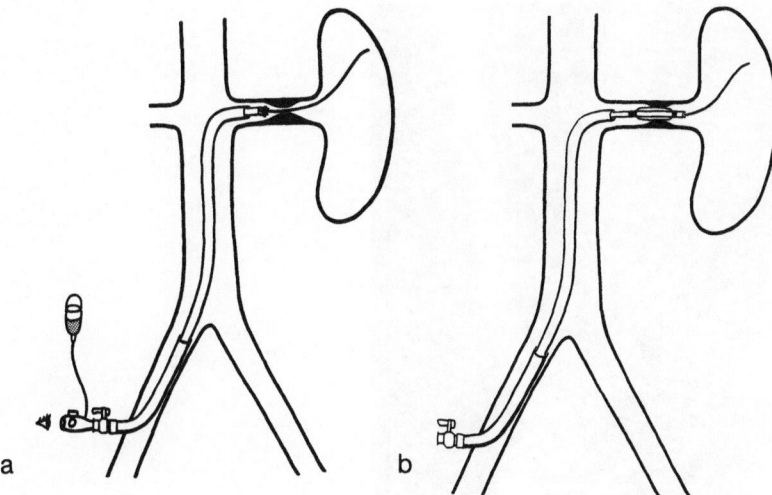

Fig. 5.2 a, b. Angioscopic control before renal artery dilation. **a** Positioning of the guide wire into the stenosed renal artery. **b** Dilatation of the stenosis by a 5-F balloon catheter introduced through the guide catheter

Fig. 5.3. Angioscopic control of the outcome of renal artery dilatation. The balloon catheter is removed; leaving the guide wire in place, the angioscope is advanced by the Seldinger technique

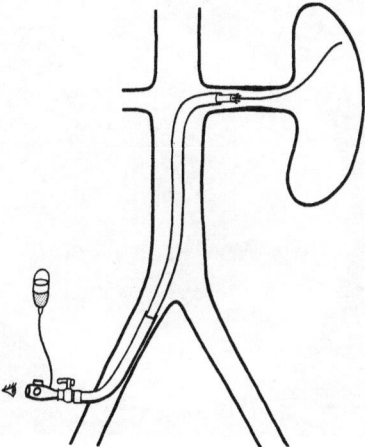

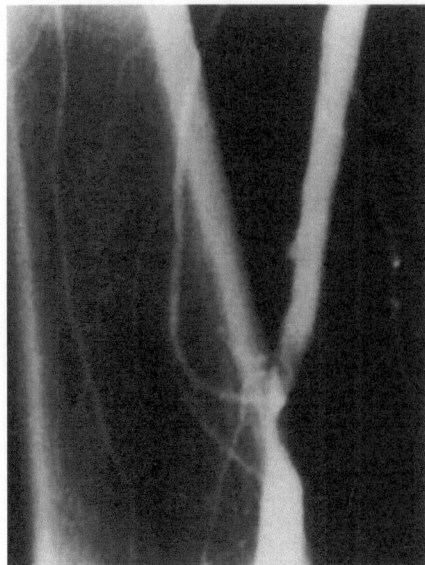

Fig. 5.4. Angiography of a high-grade stenosis of the femoral artery prior to dilatation

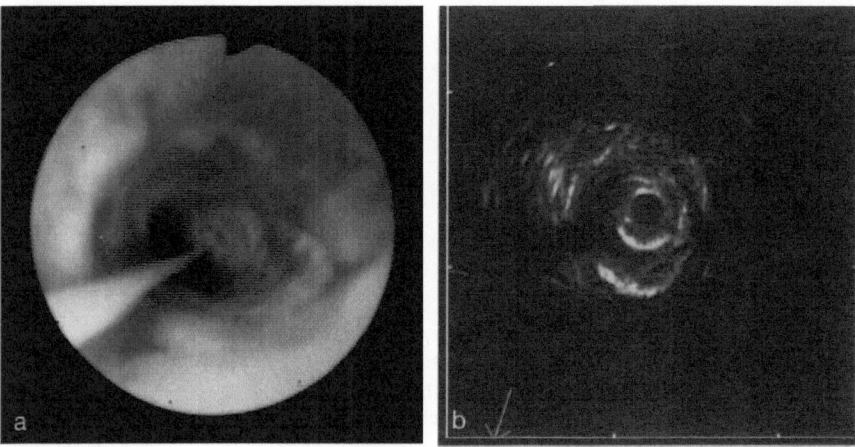

Fig. 5.5. a Angioscopy of the same vascular area as in Fig. 5.4. High-grade stenosis with multiple flat atherosclerotic plaques. **b** This endovascular picture corresponding to **a** shows a calcified stenosis with smooth material on the vessel wall

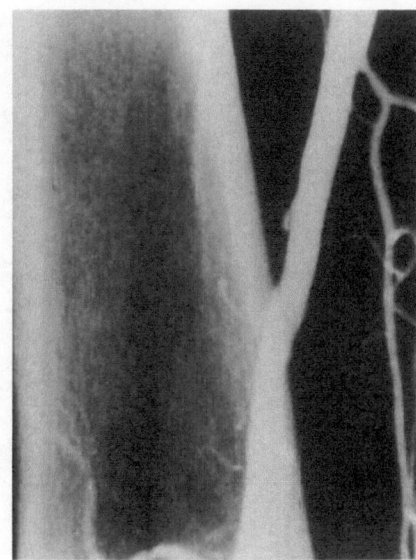

Fig. 5.6. Result of the dilatation with marked improvement and only little residual stenosis

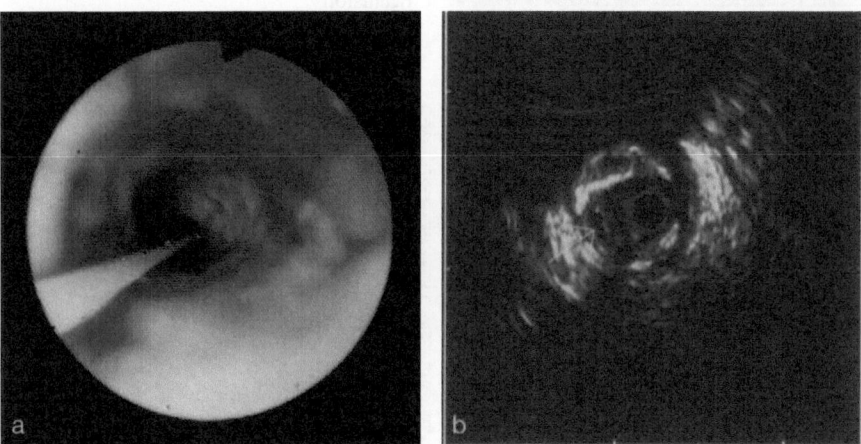

Fig. 5.7. a Angioscopic control after dilatation: only little improvement. **b** The atherosclerotic plaques are cracked and intimal flaps narrow the lumen eccentrically

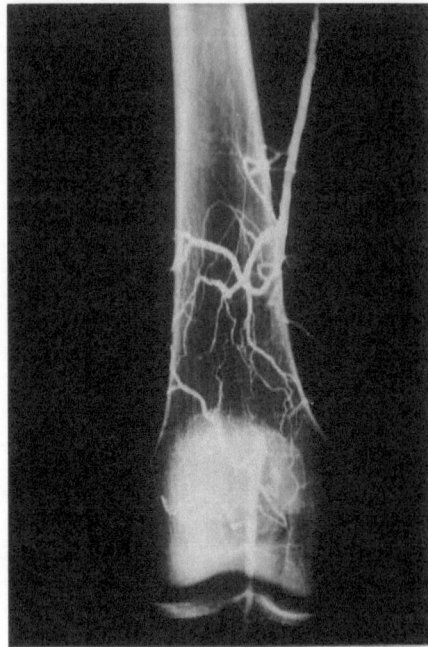

Fig. 5.8. Arteriogram of a femoral artery occlusion

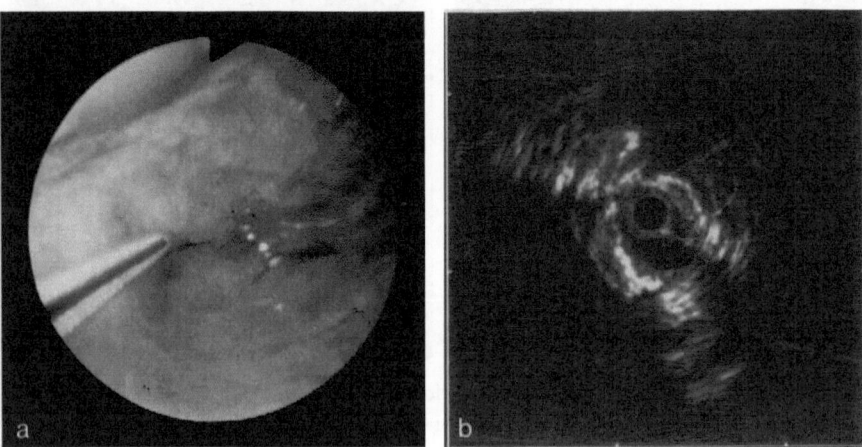

Fig. 5.9. a Angioscopy of the same femoral artery as in Fig. 5.8. The stenosis has been crossed by a guide wire. **b** Occlusion of the femoral artery seen by endovascular ultrasound. The circular stenosis is caused by an atherosclerotic calcification

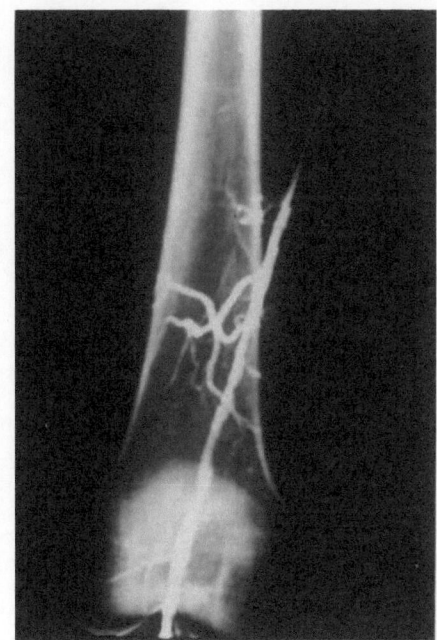

Fig. 5.10. Outcome of PTA of the femoral artery stenosis. Successful recanalization of the vessel

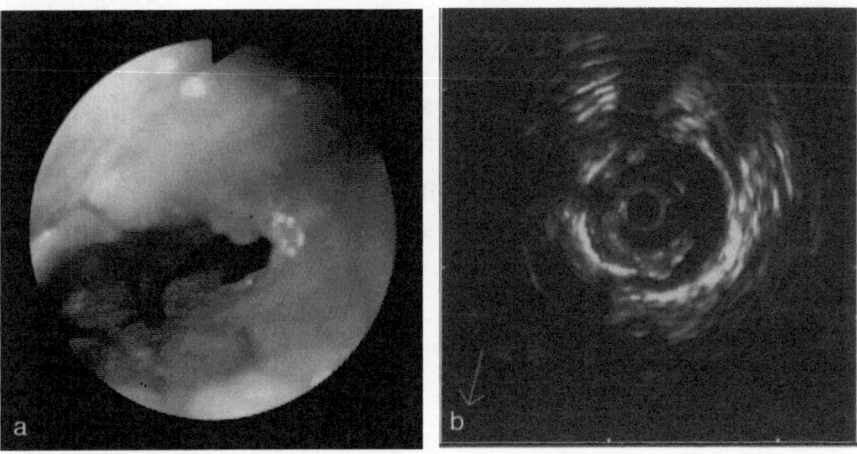

Fig. 5.11. a Eccentric vascular lumen with tears of atherosclerotic plaques. **b** After dilatation the arteriosclerotic wall is widened. The former circular stenosing plaque is divided into two parts at 11 o'clock and 5 o'clock. There is a small dissection area at 8 o'clock

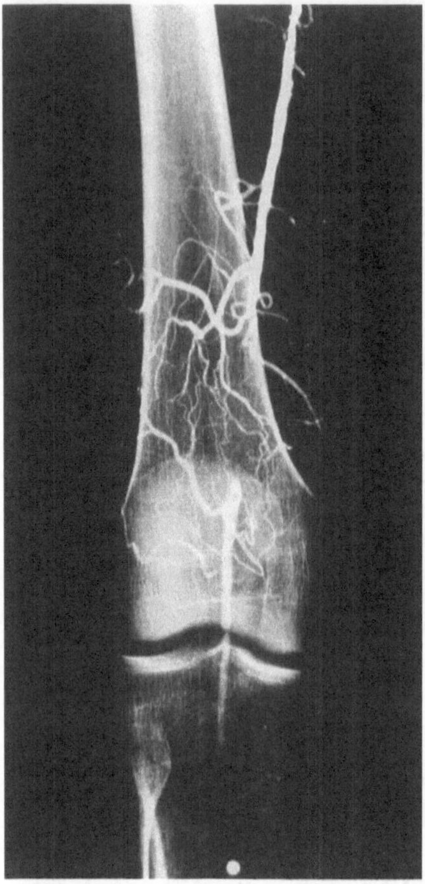

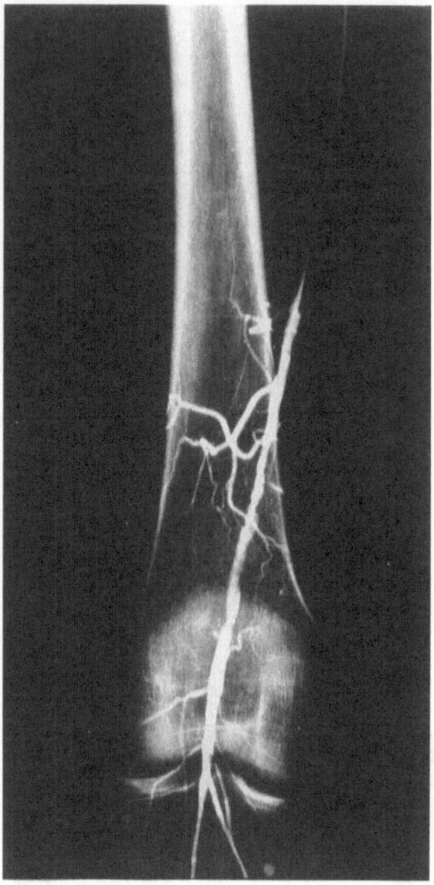

Fig. 5.12 (*left*). Atherosclerotic occlusion of the femoral artery

Fig. 5.13 (*right*). Same vessel as in Fig. 5.12 after successful dilatation

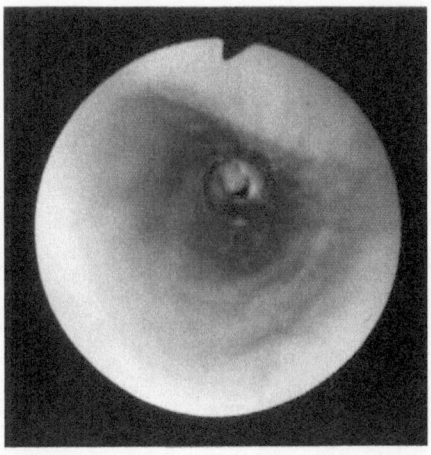 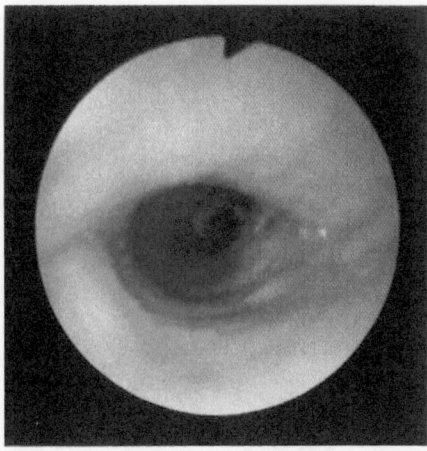

Fig. 5.14 *(left)*. Angioscopy before PTA. Atherosclerotic stenosis of the lumen

Fig. 5.15 *(right)*. Angioscopy after PTA. Opening of the plaque; irregular vascular lumen

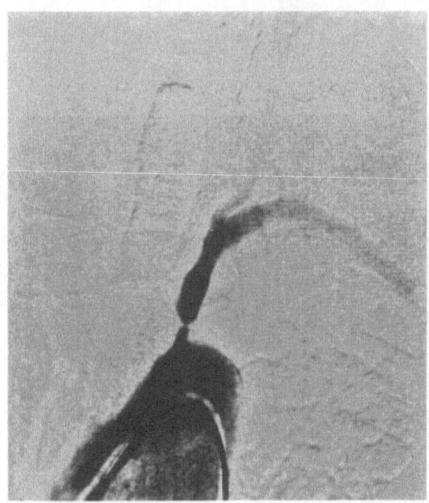

Fig. 5.16. Angiogram of a stenosis of the left subclavian artery

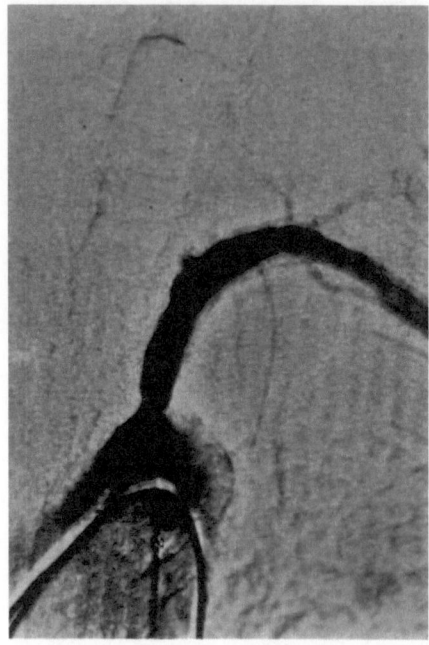

Fig. 5.17. Result after PTA with good angiographic and clinical result

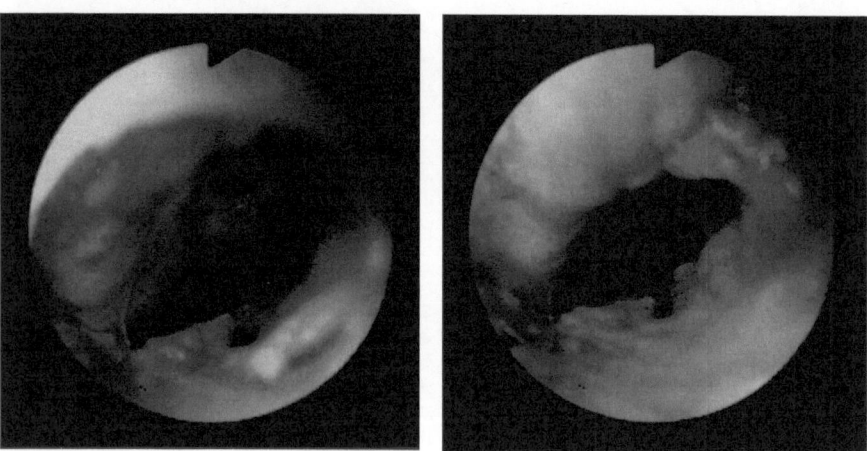

Fig. 5.18 (*left*). Angioscopic confirmation of severe atherosclerosis with eccentric vascular lumen

Fig. 5.19 (*right*). Result of PTA of the subclavian stenosis with distinct tear of the atherosclerotic plaques

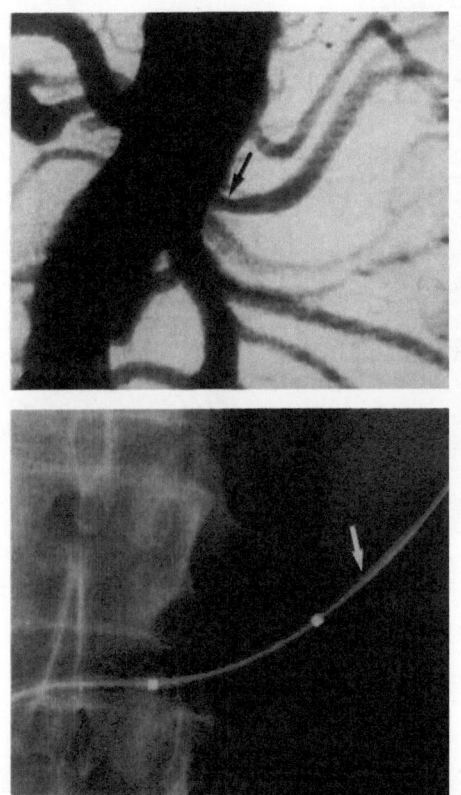

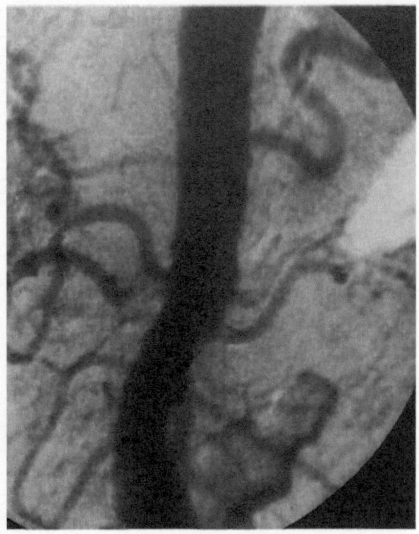

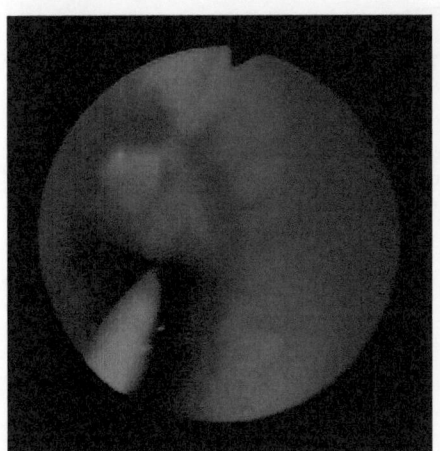

Fig. 5.20 (*upper left*). High-grade renal artery stenosis with plaque at the aortic origin

Fig. 5.21 (*lower left*). Technical procedure: guide catheter (*arrow*), dilatation catheter, and guide wire

Fig. 5.22 (*right*). Result of successful PTA with residual stenosis and minor dissection

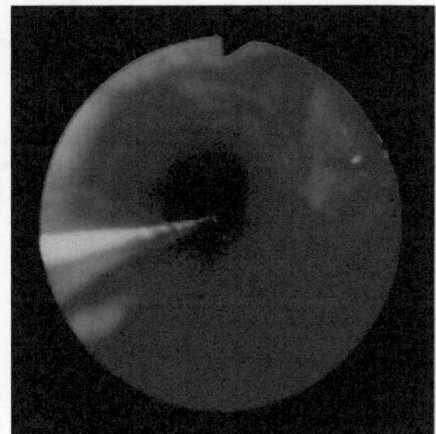

Fig. 5.23 (*left*). Renal artery stenosis with eccentric plaque

Fig. 5.24 (*right*). Result after successful PTA. The stenosis is markedly dilated; circular intimal tears

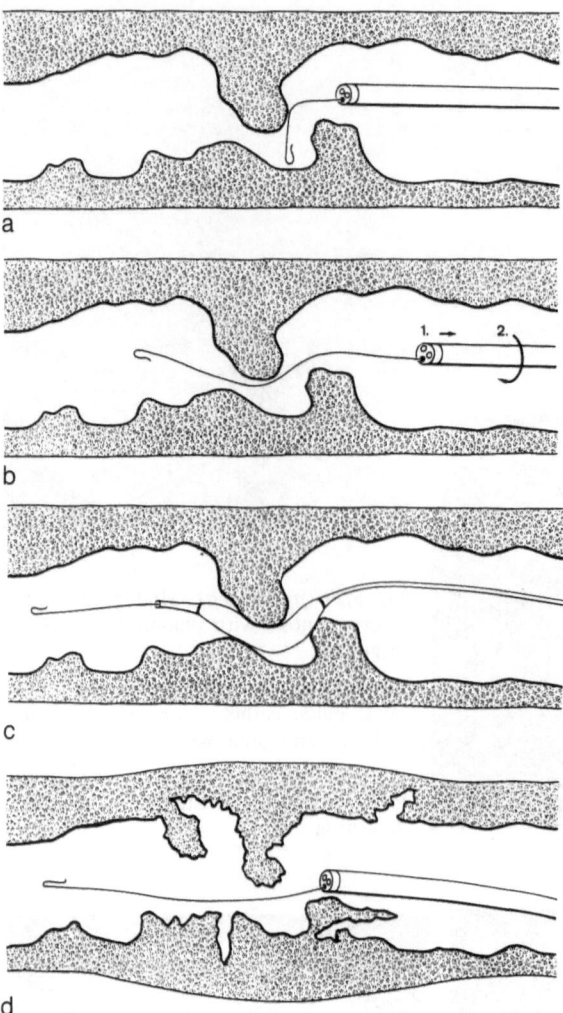

Fig. 5.25. a Angioscopy of a stenosis that can usually not be crossed. **b** In many cases a way can be found by pulling back and turning the angioscope. **c** Conventional balloon catheter dilatation. **d** On advancing the angioscope to the dilated vascular region the vascular damage with typical "cracks" can be seen

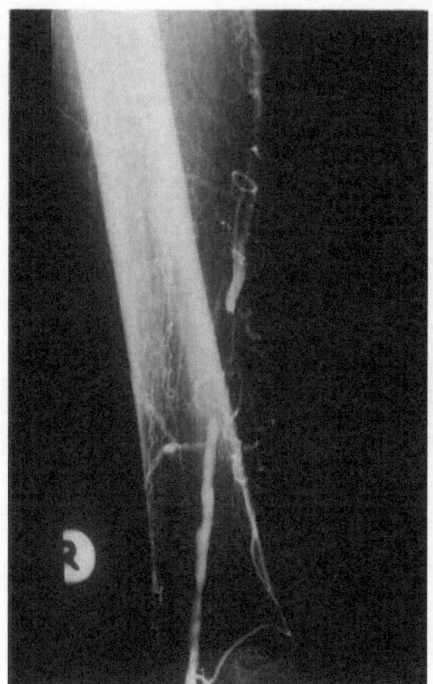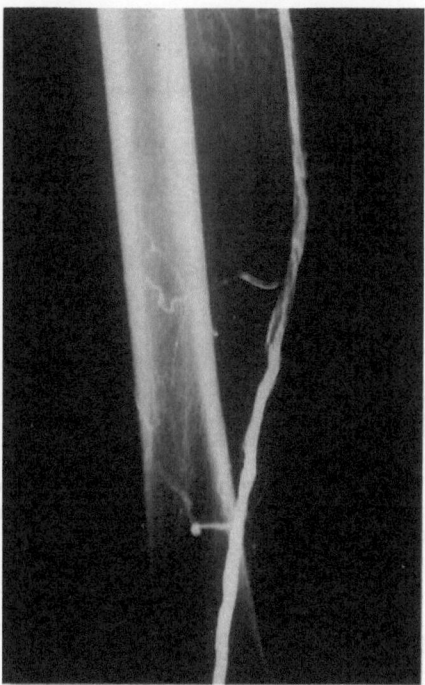

Fig. 5.26 (*left*). Thrombotic occlusion of the femoral artery by fresh thrombi

Fig. 5.27 (*right*). Result of local thrombolysis and dilatation with confirmation of a mural thrombosis

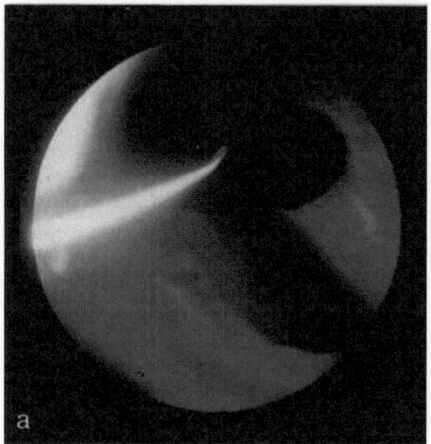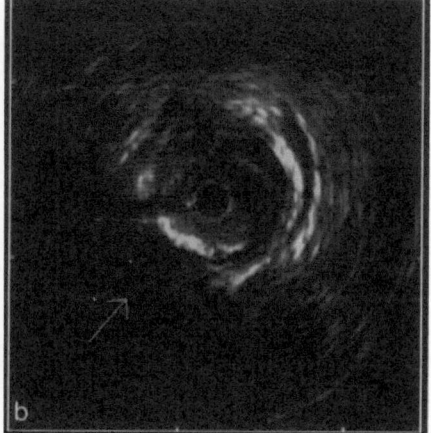

Fig. 5.28. a Thrombotic occlusion with additional mural thrombosis. **b** Thrombotic lesion of the femoral artery. The endovascular ultrasound shows a hypodense thrombotic area around the catheter tip which passed the lesion. Atherosclerosis of the vessel wall is indicated by the *arrow*

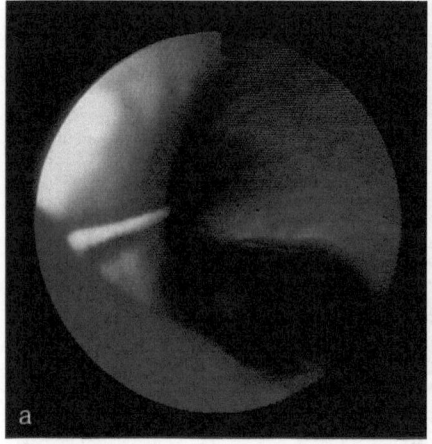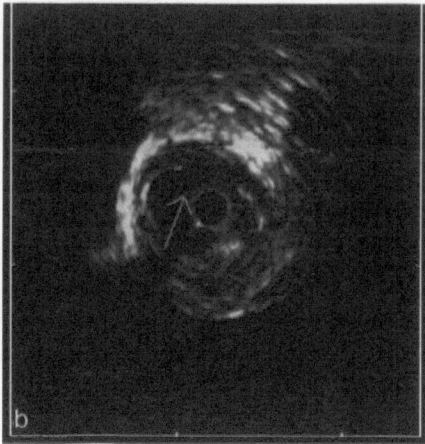

Fig. 5.29. a Outcome of local thrombolysis and dilatation with residual thrombus. **b** After local lysis the arterial lumen is partially recanalized. The patent part of the lumen (*arrow*) is slit-shaped

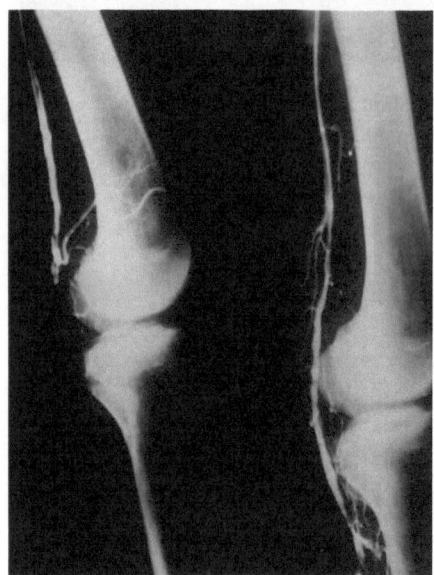

Fig. 5.30. A 75-year-old patient with embolic occlusion of the right popliteal artery (*left*). *Right*, result after successful local catheter lysis with a total dose of 850 000 U urokinase administered through an angioscope

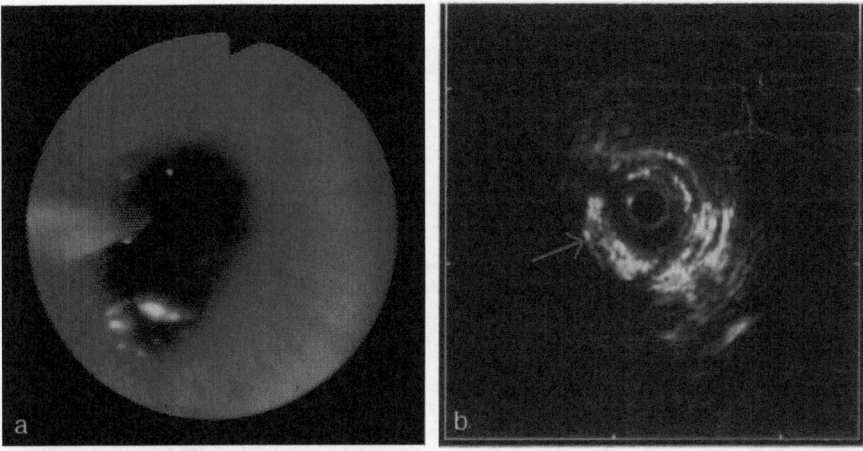

Fig. 5.31. a The same patient as in Fig. 5.30, with occlusion of the popliteal artery seen by angioscopy. The surface of the thrombus is perforated by the guide wire. **b** Calcified arteriosclerotic and thrombotic occlusion of the femoral artery (*arrow*) with multiple hyperdense narrowing plaques diagnosed by endovascular ultrasound

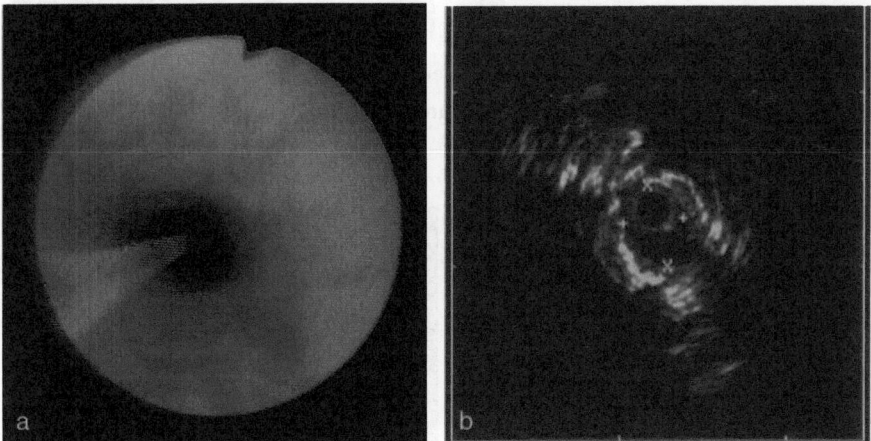

Fig. 5.32. a Result of local thrombolysis with a total dose of 850 000 U urokinase. An additional atherosclerotic plaque is revealed. **b** The result of local lysis and subsequent balloon dilatation is evident: the calcifications of the vessel wall became more dense and the lumen is patent (measurement of patency: from × to ×, 7 mm; from + to + 4 mm)

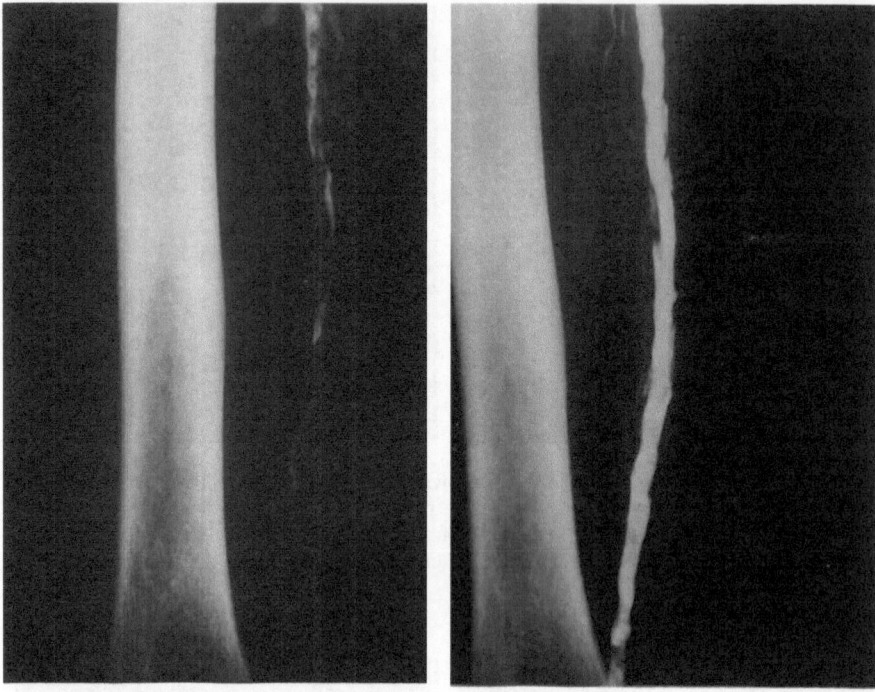

Fig. 5.33 (*left*). Occlusion of the femoral superficial artery by intravascular thrombosis

Fig. 5.34 (*right*). Result of successful local thrombolysis with residual thrombosis

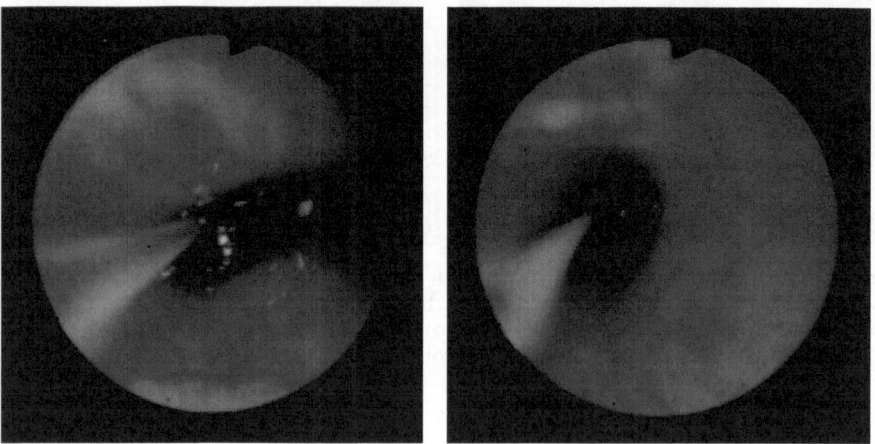

Fig. 5.35. Local thrombosis of the superficial femoral artery with atherosclerosis

Fig. 5.36. Result of successful thrombolysis with residual thrombosis and additional atherosclerosis

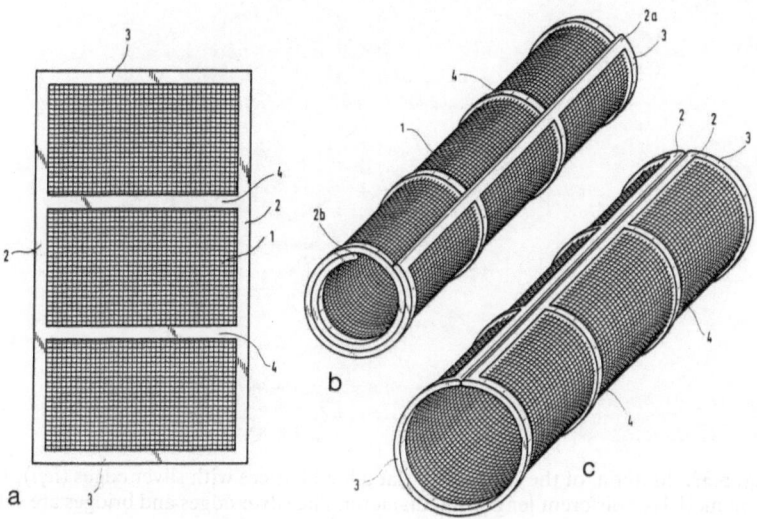

Fig. 5.37a–c. Diagram of the endoprosthesis. **a** Lattice is made from gilded brass wires, 0.14 mm thick (*1*). The longitudinal edges (*2*), transverse edges (*3*), and two cross-pieces (*4*) of the lattice are enclosed with silver for better elasticity. **b** The lattice in its compressed condition. The lattice (*1*) is wrapped 1.5 times around the balloon catheter. It expands to three times the size after dilatation. The cross-pieces (*4*) expand as well and ensure stability (*2a, 2b*). **c** The lattice (*1*) in the dilated condition. The longitudinal silver edges (*2*) are lined up and prevent the collapse of the stent when the balloon catheter is removed (the so-called elastic recoiling)

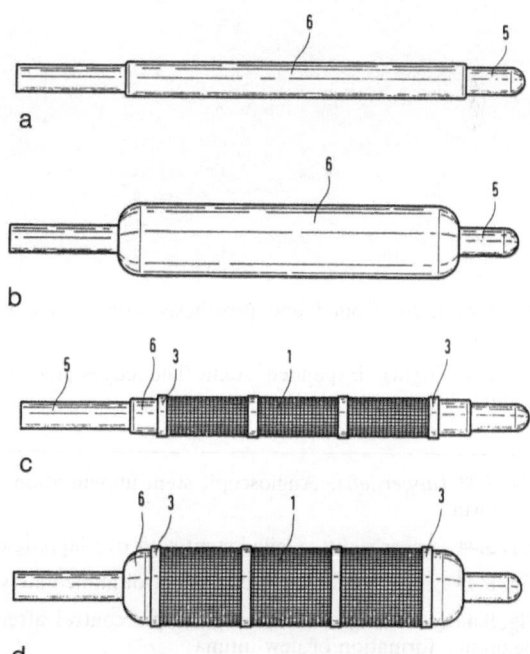

Fig. 5.38a–d. Diagram of the mechanism of stent dilatation. **a** A 7-F balloon catheter not inflated (*6*). **b** The same balloon catheter inflated. **c** The endoprosthesis is placed on the non-inflated balloon catheter (*3, 1*). **d** Dilated balloon and endoprosthesis

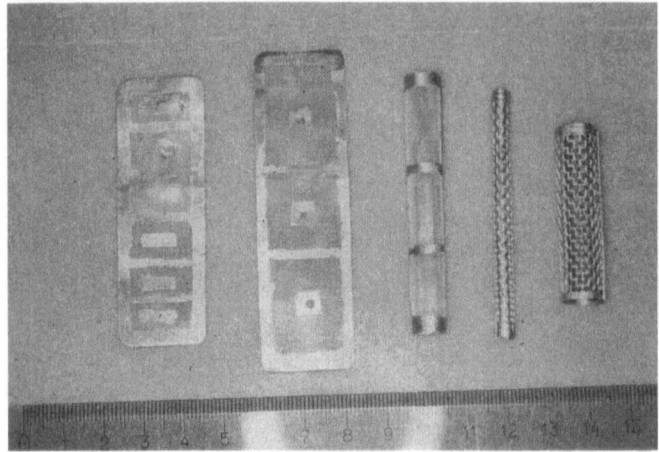

Fig. 5.39. Material of the stents. Two flat gilded lattices with silver edges (*left*). Expanded stent models of different length and diameter. The silver edges and bridges are soldered for stability

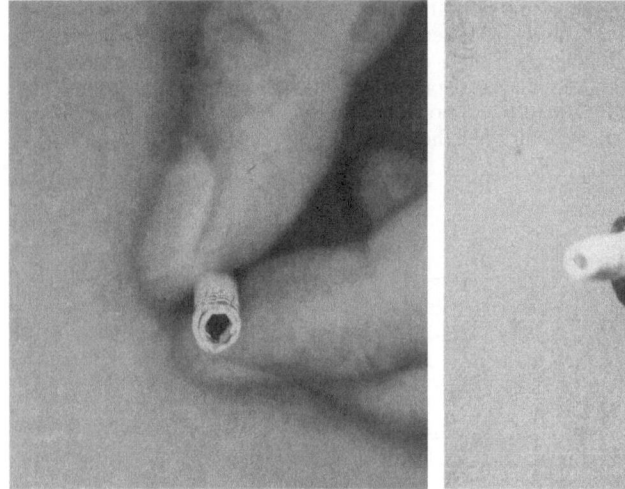

Fig. 5.40 (*left*). Coiled endoprosthesis with double winding. The outside diameter is 2.1 mm

Fig. 5.41 (*right*). Expanded stent. The edges line up. The outside diameter is now 8 mm

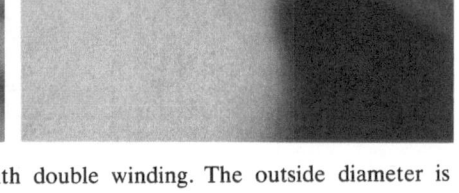

Fig. 5.43 (*upper left*). Angioscopic stent implantation. The coiled stent is advanced into the aorta

Fig. 5.44 (*upper right*). Coiled stent with overlapping edges

Fig. 5.45 (*lower left*). Angioscopic control immediately after stent implantation

Fig. 5.46 (*lower right*). Late angioscopic control after 8 weeks of stent implantation. Beginning formation of new intima

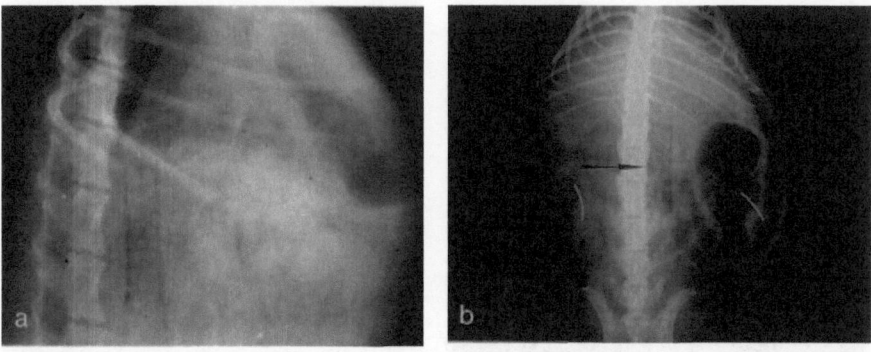

Fig. 5.42. a Stent implantation into the abdominal aorta of a dog. The endoprosthesis was followed-up for 8 months and was tolerated by the dog without complication. **b** Implantation of a stent into the aorta of a rat. The stent had been tolerated for 12 months without any complications (modified Beck stent with plastic surface)

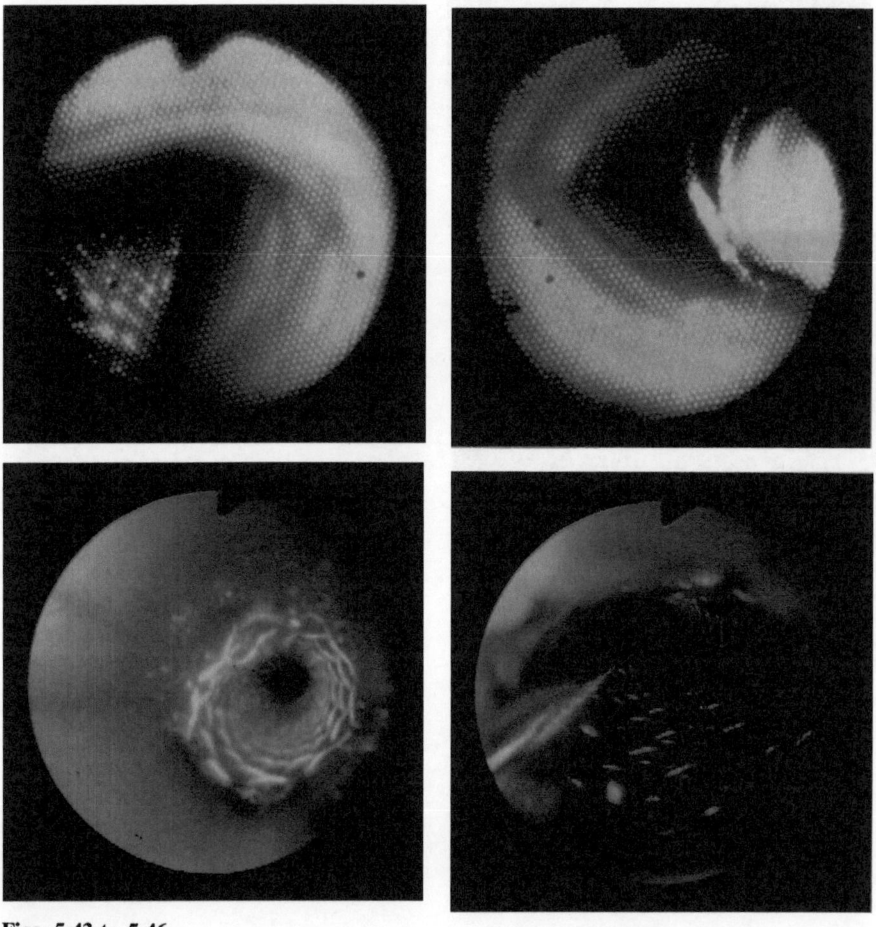

Figs. 5.43 to 5.46

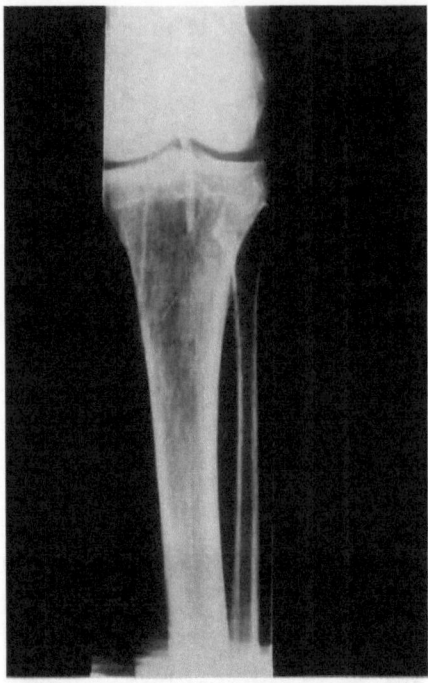

Fig. 5.47. A 68-year-old patient with occlusion of the popliteal artery. Development of collateral arteries over sural branches. Distal vessels are only barely outlined

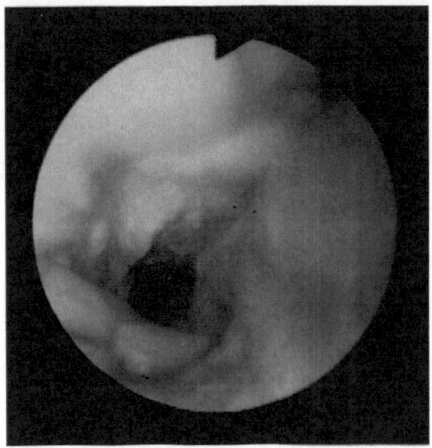

Fig. 5.48. Angioscopic severe atherosclerosis with high-grade stenosing plaques directly proximal to the occlusion

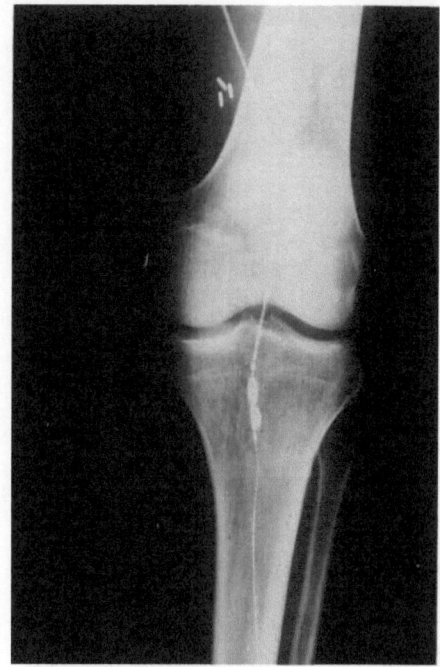

Fig. 5.49. The same patient as in Fig. 5.48. Attempt to dilate the occlusion; the balloon cannot be completely inflated because of the rigidity of the atherosclerotic plaque

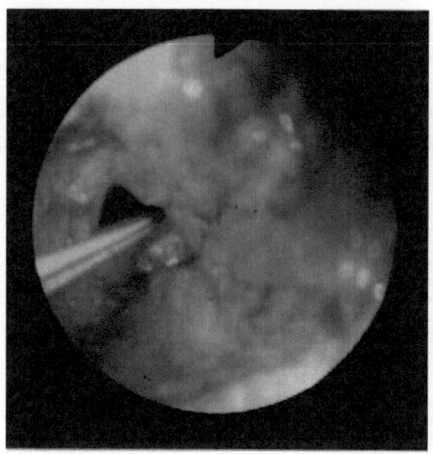

Fig. 5.50. Only minor success after dilatation. High-grade residual stenosis. The guide wire is advanced through the dilated vascular region

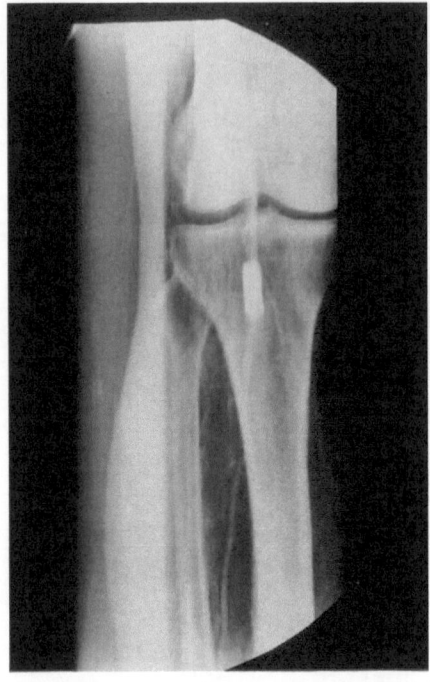

Fig. 5.51. Result of percutaneous stent implantation without flow disturbances of contrast medium. No stenosis of the stent can be detected by angiography

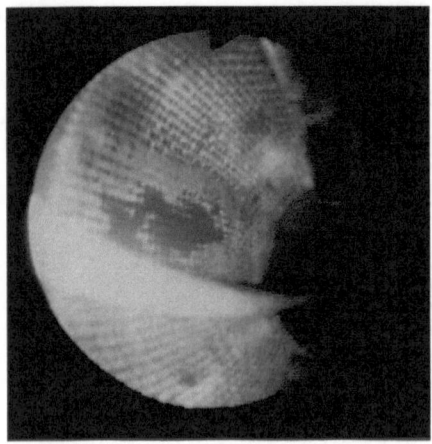

Fig. 5.52. Wide open vessel immediately after stent implantation detected by angioscopy. Minor thrombotic, wall-adherent depositions on the inside surface of the stent

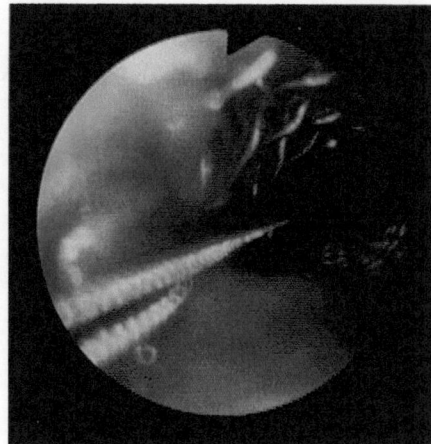

Fig. 5.53. The same patient as in Fig. 5.52, 3 months after stent implantation. Angioscopic view through the stent with view of the popliteal artery. Parts of the metal are already covered by vascular wall tissue

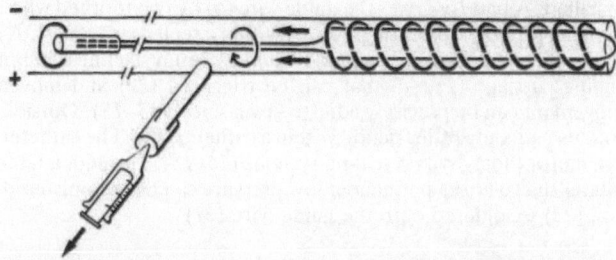

Fig. 5.54. Simplified diagram of the principle of percutaneous thrombus extraction. With constant suction and continuous drilling thrombotic material is aspirated into the catheter where it is cut into pieces and removed from the catheter

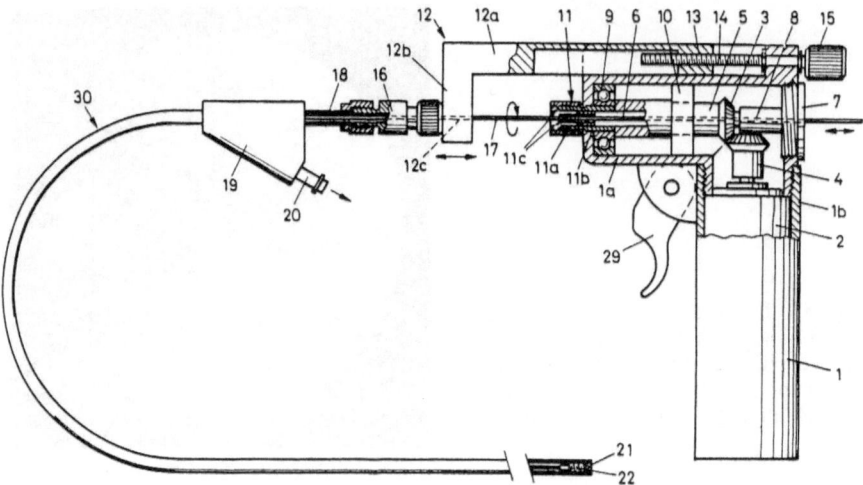

Fig. 5.55. Technical diagram of the thrombus extraction device. Within the handle (*1*) of the pistol-shaped device (polyurethane surface; *1a, 1b*) a 12-V direct-current motor (*2*) is installed. A battery drives the guide wire (*6*) by two toothed wheels (*4, 5*). The guide wire is kept in place by two bearings (*9, 10*) within a sealed system (*7*). A sleeve (*11*) keeps the wire in the correct position. The guide wire has 2-mm slackness in both directions assured by a sliding carriage (*11a–c*) that can be triggered (*29*) and moved on a bar (*12a–c*). This movement can be precisely adjusted by a screw (*13–15*). Outside the motor the guide wire rotates with only little friction within a catheter (*30*). The catheter itself is firmly attached to the motor block by two sealing systems (*16, 18*). Through a lateral safety valve (*19*) and a lateral sleeve (*20*) a permanent low pressure can be administered. Within the catheter tip a coil (*22*) is soldered onto the guide wire (*21*)

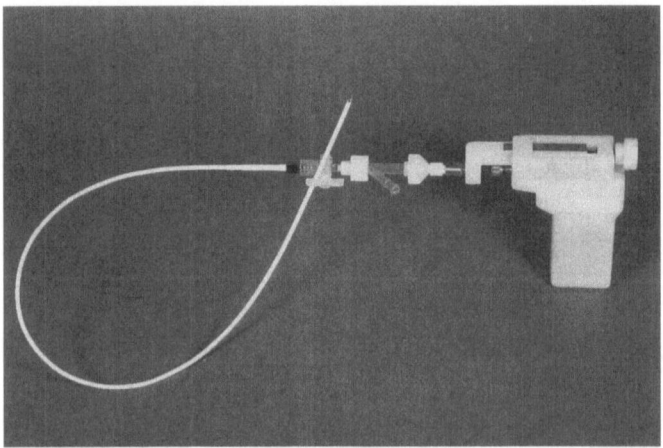

Fig. 5.56. The thrombus extraction device. A direct-current motor of 12 V with a variable speed of transmission from 15 to 20 000 RPM is attached to the handle. The rotation of the wire is transmitted by a shaft. When triggering, the wire is moved within the catheter so that the thrombotic material can be easily aspirated and removed

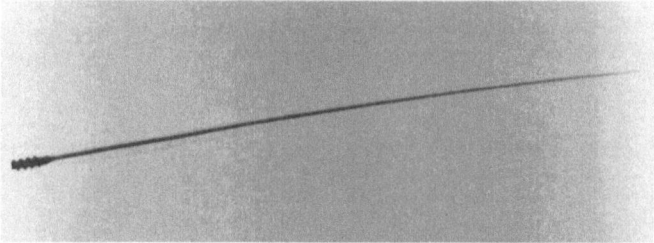

Fig. 5.57. X-ray of the thrombus extraction catheter. The visible drilling coil at the tip of the guide wire is enclosed by the catheter. The drilling tip remains within the catheter during thrombus extraction

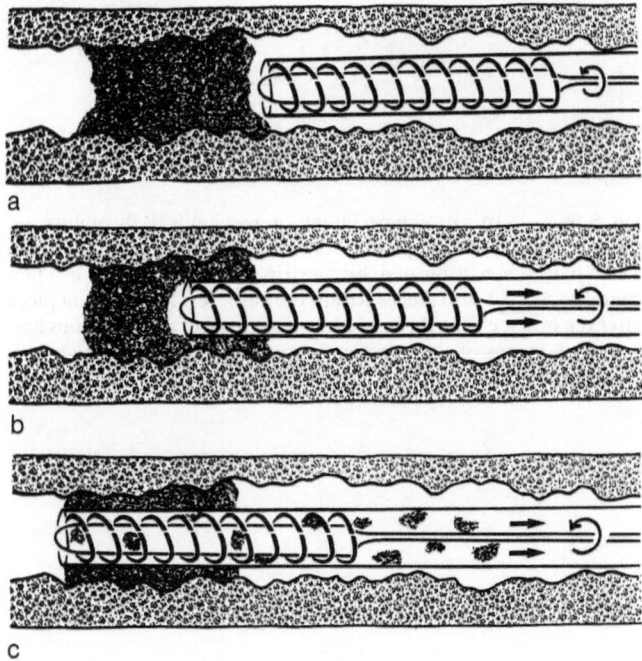

Fig. 5.58 a–c. Diagram of the three steps of thrombus extraction. **a** The catheter with the drilling device is positioned just in front of the thrombus. **b** The thrombus is aspirated and simultaneously cut into pieces. **c** After aspiration the vascular lumen is open

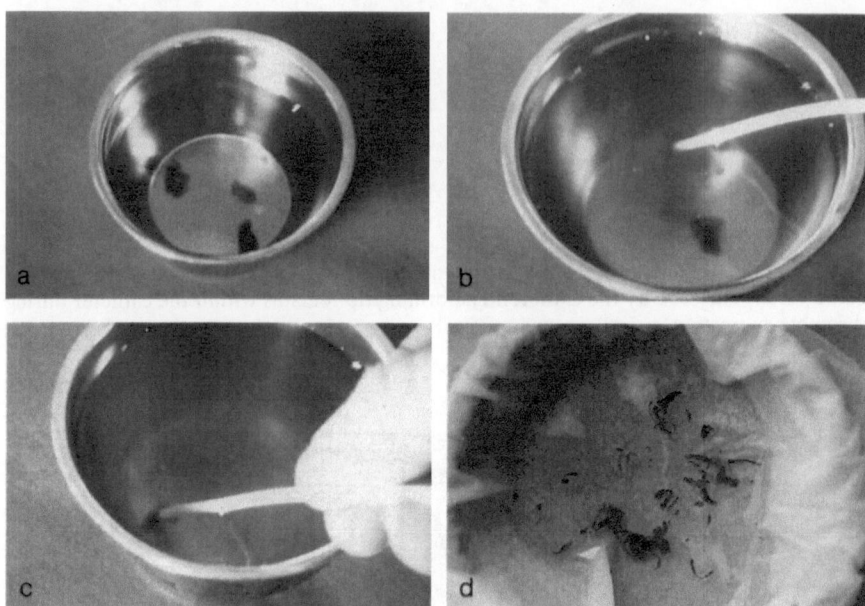

Fig. 5.59 a–c. In vitro experiment of mechanical thrombus extraction. **a** Two human thrombi, each measuring 3 cm in diameter, float in a physiological sodium chloride solution. They have been aspirated by the tip of the catheter. **b** Thereafter, the thrombus is continuously cut into pieces within the catheter. The residual pieces are then aspirated one after the other. **c** The thrombi are aspirated after the thrombus has been completely cut into pieces. **d** Pieces of thrombotic material that were aspirated through the catheter

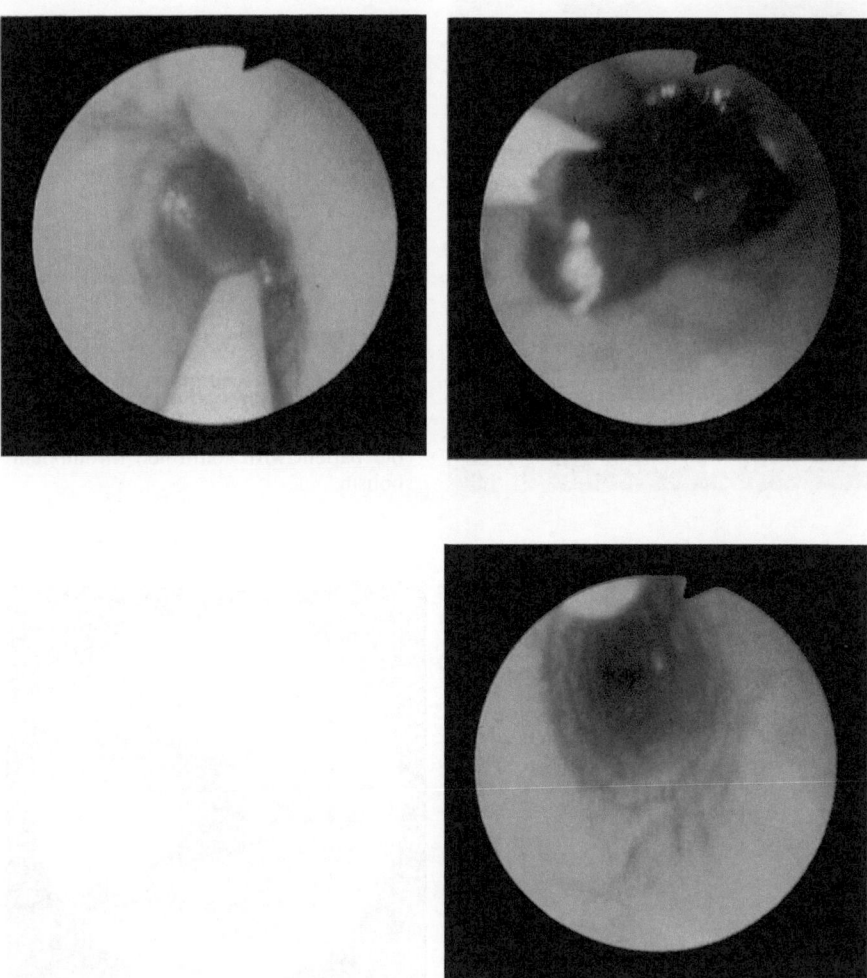

Fig. 5.60 (*upper left*). Angioscopically confirmed large thrombus in the iliac artery of a dog

Fig. 5.61 (*upper right*). Aspirated thrombus at the catheter tip

Fig. 5.62 (*lower right*). Result of complete thrombus extraction without local thrombolysis in a dog. The manipulation by the thrombus extraction device has not injured the vessel

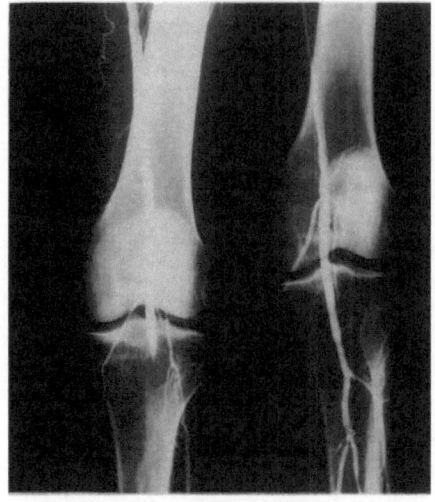

Fig. 5.63. Acute occlusion of the popliteal artery (*left*) and the outcome of thrombus extraction (*right*) in a 70-year-old patient with confirmed thromboembolism

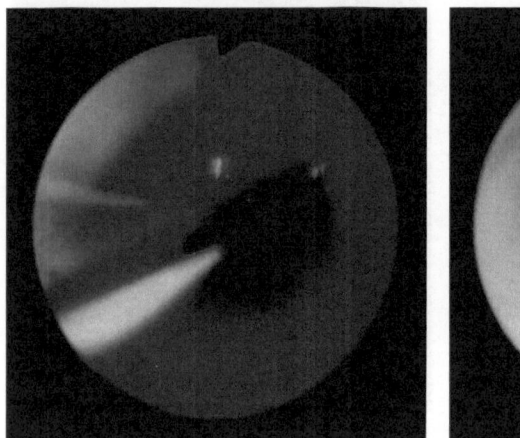

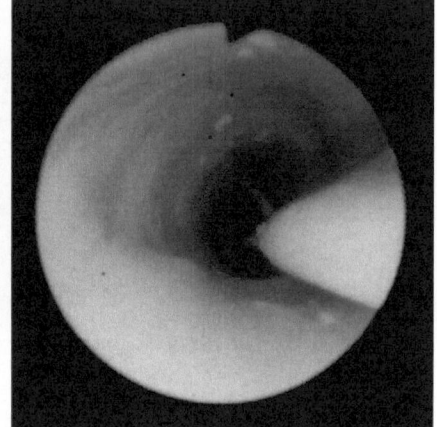

Fig. 5.64 (*left*). Thromboembolic vascular occlusion of the popliteal artery. The guide wire runs through the mural thrombus

Fig. 5.65 (*right*). Result of successful thrombus extraction. Evidence of atherosclerosis. The photograph shows a free guide wire

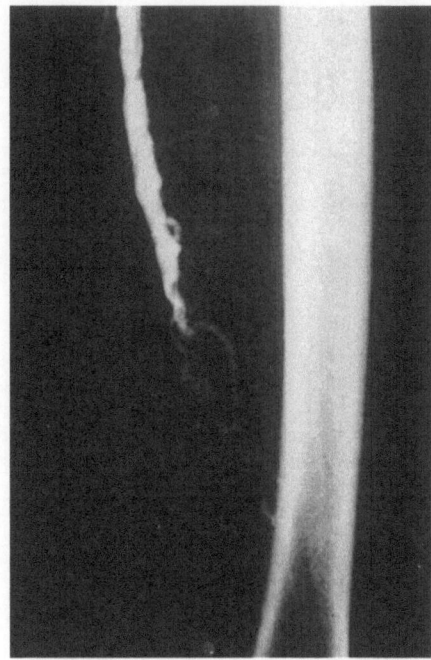

Fig. 5.66. Long stenosis of the femoral artery. A local lysis was unsuccessful

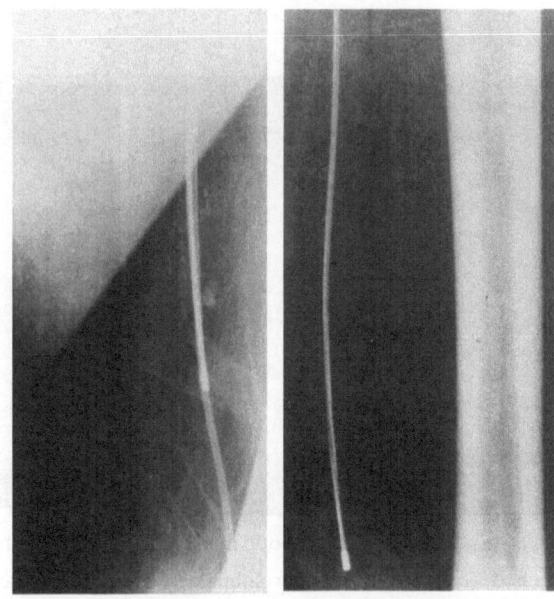

Fig. 5.67 (*left*). Advancing a 7-F catheter distally to the thrombus. The coil is located at the middle third of the catheter

Fig. 5.68 (*right*). The catheter with the coil has reached the thrombus

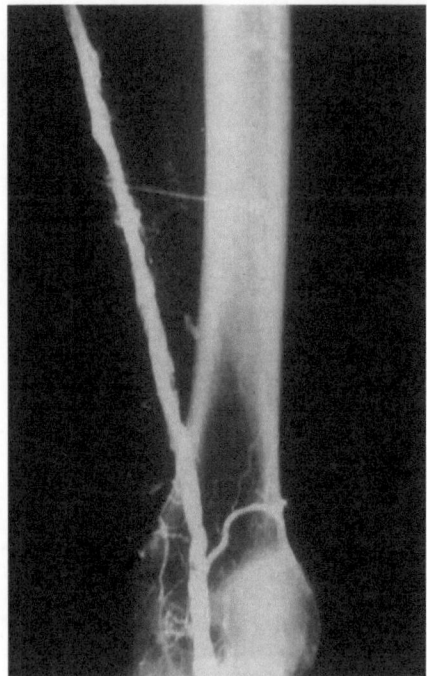

Fig. 5.69. Successful thrombus extraction with good run-off of contrast medium to the periphery

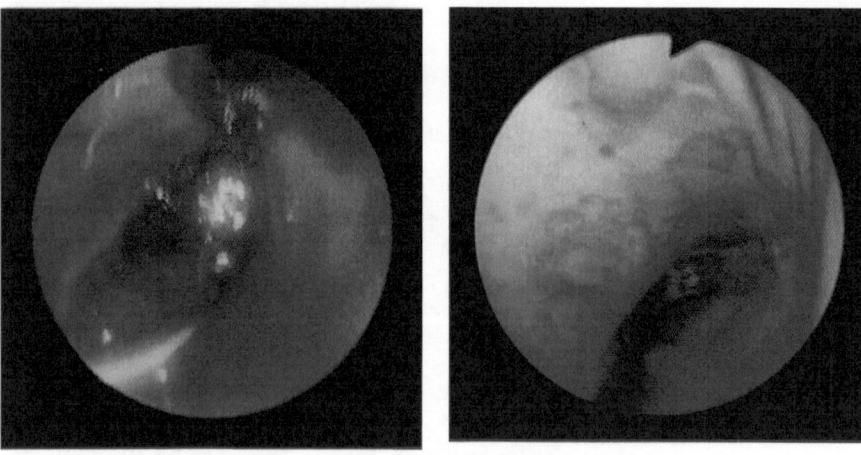

Fig. 5.70 (*left*). Fresh thrombotic material occluding the femoral artery

Fig. 5.71 (*right*). Result of thrombus extraction. Atherosclerosis

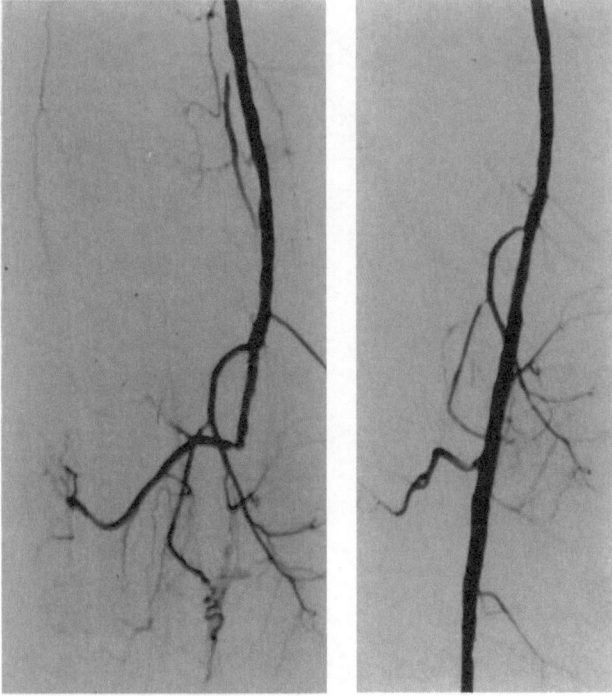

Fig. 5.72 *(left)*. Arteriogram of an occluded femoral artery. Local lysis was not indicated because of the risk of bleeding in hypocoagulability

Fig. 5.73 *(right)*. Situation of the same patient after percutaneous transluminal thrombectomy and final dilatation. The artery is patent

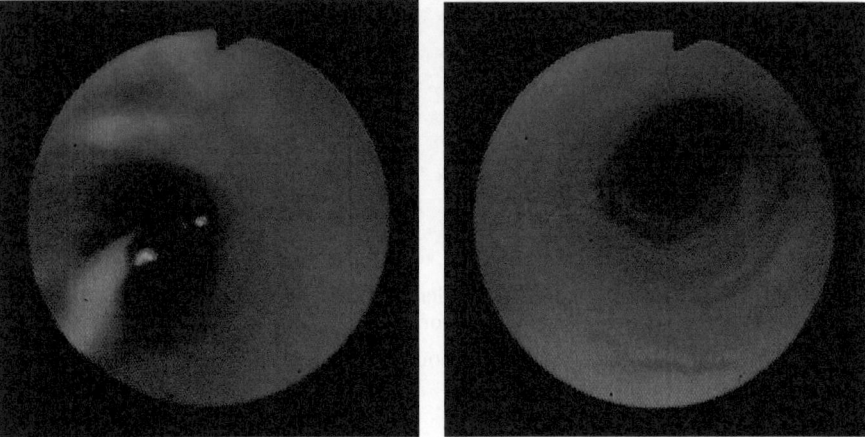

Fig. 5.74 *(left)*. Occlusion of a femoral artery. Angiographically, an occluding embolus in combination with a severe arteriosclerosis can be observed

Fig. 5.75 *(right)*. The femoral artery after percutaneous thrombectomy. The patent artery shows only few alterations and lesions after the intervention

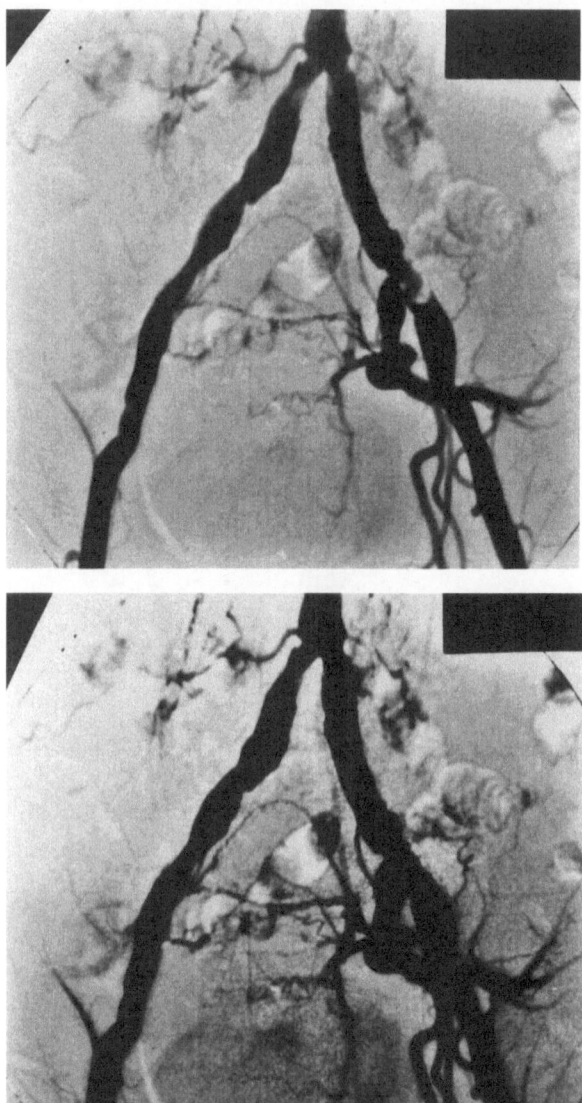

Fig. 5.76 (*above*). Thromboembolus in the iliac artery. A local lysis seemed to be too risky and a percutaneous thrombectomy was performed

Fig. 5.77 (*below*). Situation after percutaneous thrombectomy: the iliac artery is patent

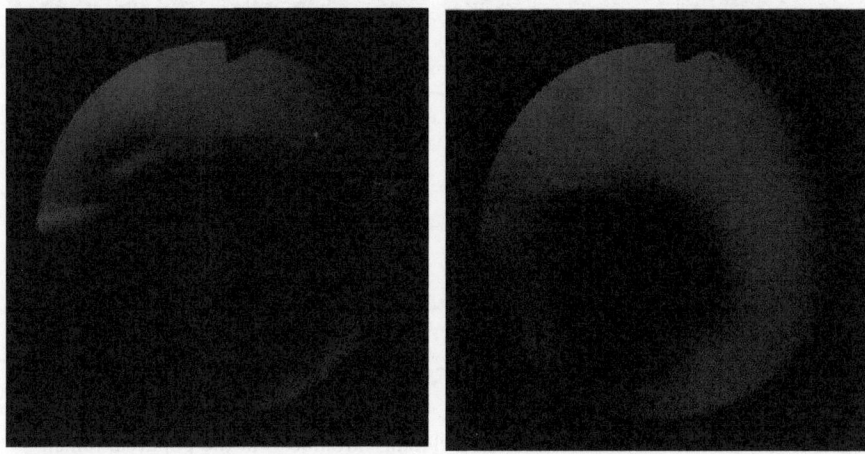

Fig. 5.78 (*left*). An occluding thrombus is situated in the iliac artery

Fig. 5.79 (*right*). After thrombectomy the patent artery shows no remarkable damage of the vessel wall

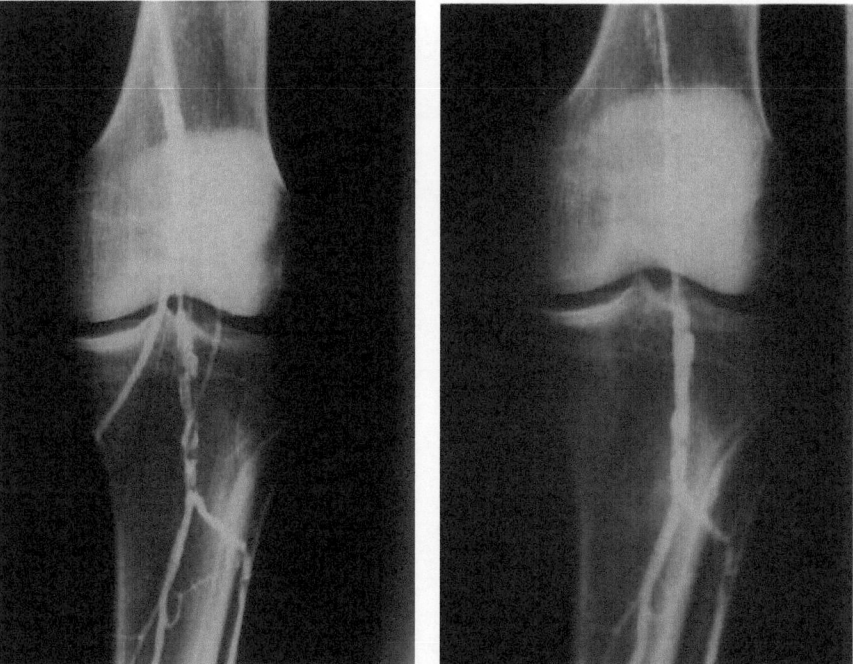

Fig. 5.80 (*left*). Thromboembolic lesion of the popliteal artery. Local lysis was not effective

Fig. 5.81 (*right*). Situation after mechanical percutaneous thrombectomy with rest: thrombotic material

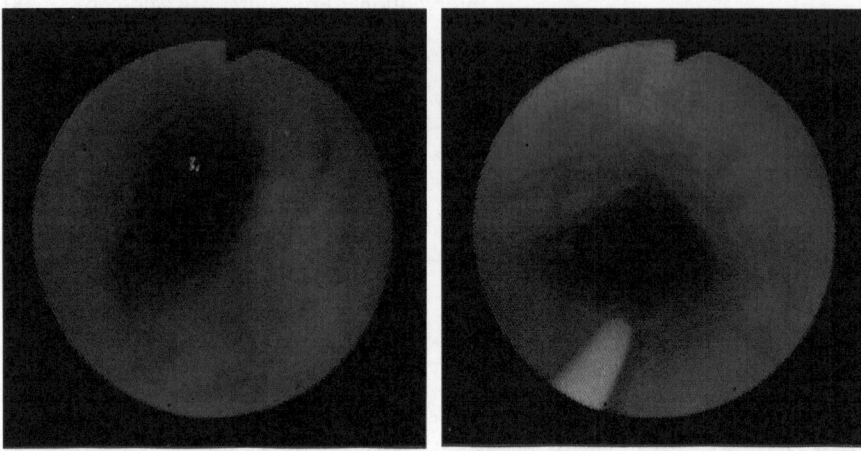

Fig. 5.82 (*left*). Arteriosclerosis with an occluding thrombosis in the popliteal lumen

Fig. 5.83 (*right*). After mechanical percutaneous thrombus extraction and a local lysis the arteriosclerotically altered vessel wall can be seen. The lumen is stenosed, corresponding to the angiographical findings

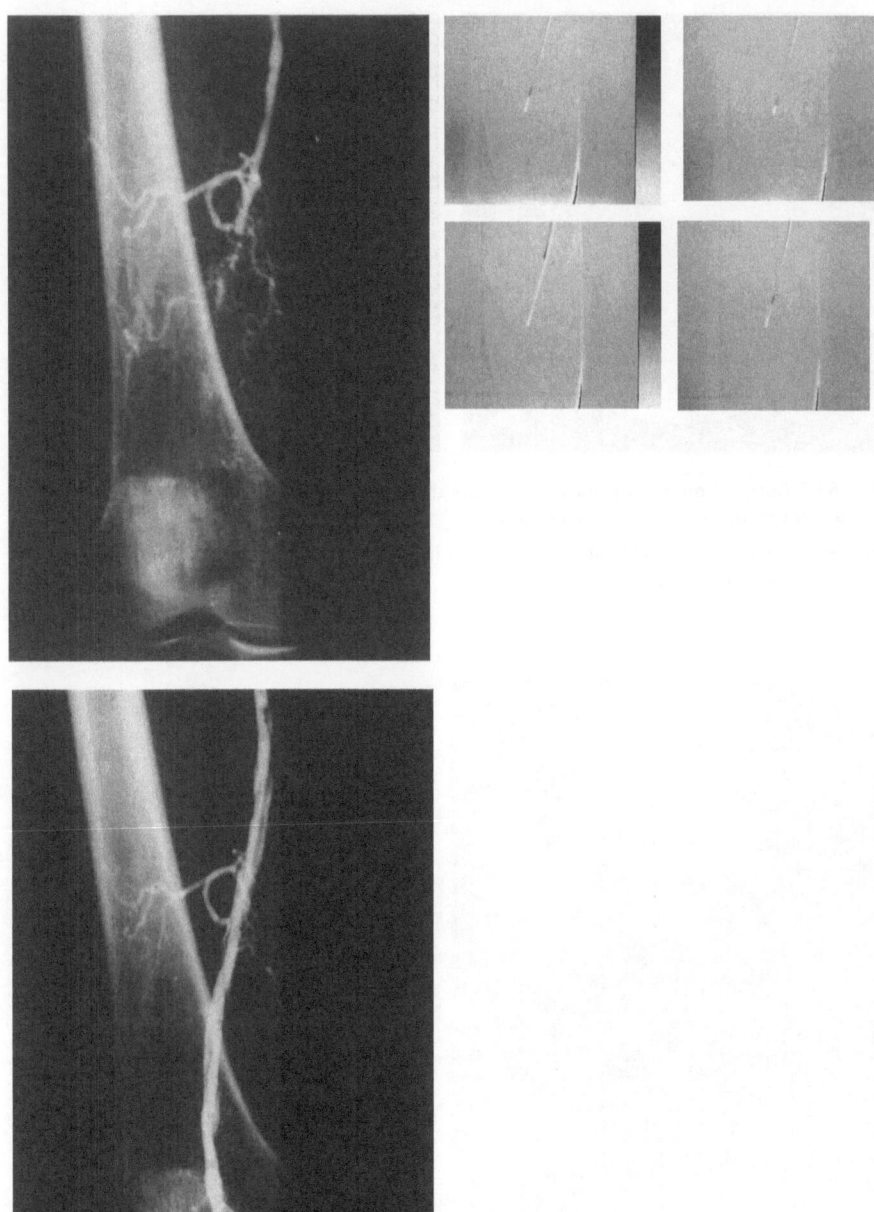

Fig. 5.84 (*upper left*). Long distant occlusion of a femoral artery. Clinical stage III

Fig. 5.85 (*upper right*). The rotation device is passing the occluded arterial segment

Fig. 5.86 (*lower left*). The artery is reopened with severe residual stenosis, wall-adherent thrombosis, and small dissections

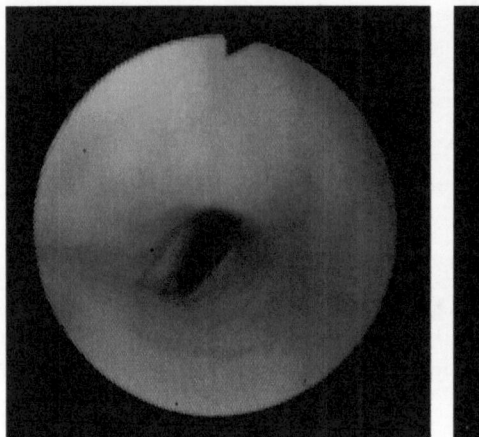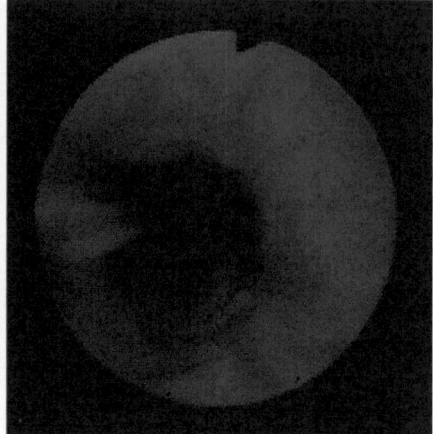

Fig. 5.87 (*left*). Angioscopy shows a remarkable stenosis caused by arteriosclerosis. The occlusion can be seen in the background

Fig. 5.88 (*right*). The rotation device in combination with a conventional dilatation shows severe lesions in the whole vessel wall

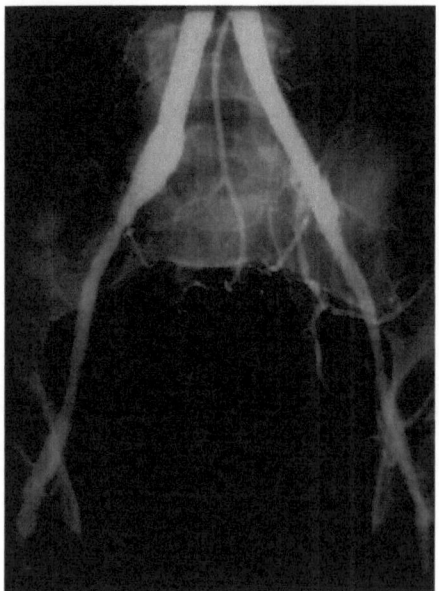

Fig. 5.89. After implantation of a Y-prosthesis the patient suffered from a stage II occlusion on the right. Angiography shows a patent iliac artery with a low-grade stenosis

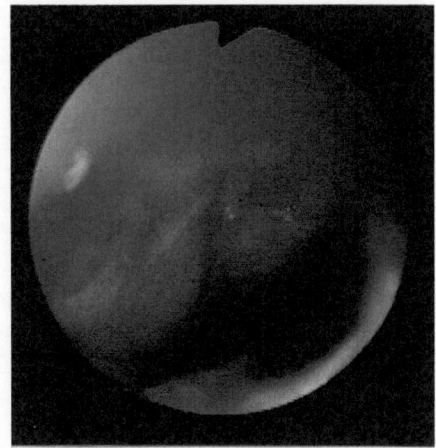

Fig. 5.90. Angioscopy of the right iliac artery revealed a slit-shaped lumen near the severe anastomosis

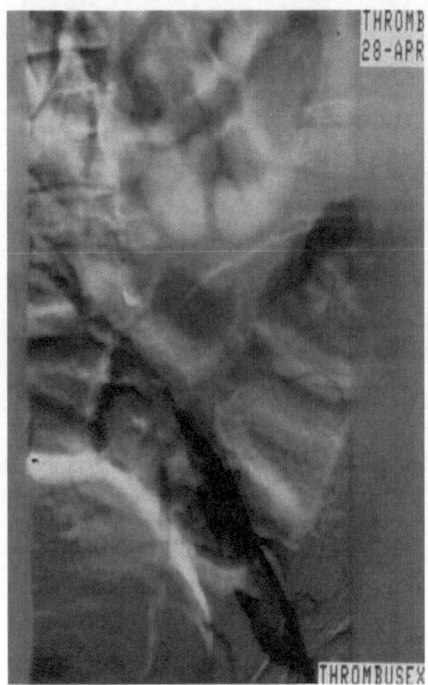

Fig. 5.91. A 17-year-old female with thrombosis in the left iliac vein. Systemic lysis was not successful

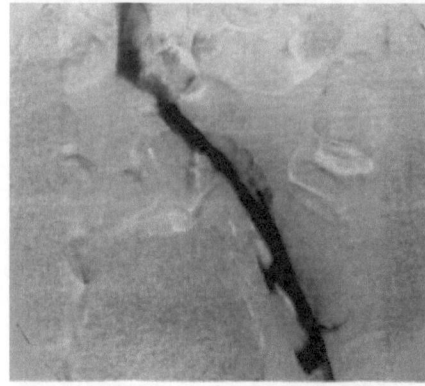

Fig. 5.92. The situation after reopening of the iliac vein by percutaneous thrombectomy. The vein wall is irregularly shaped and contains thrombotic material which could not be removed totally

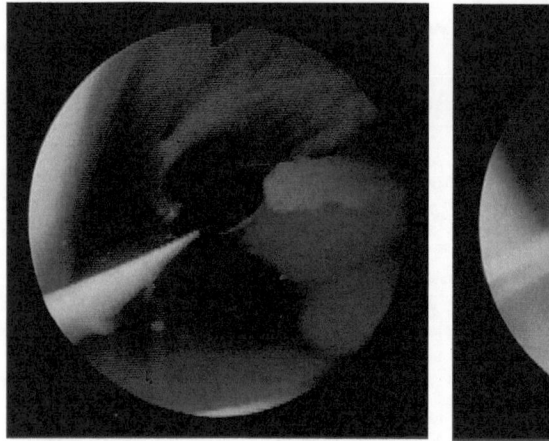

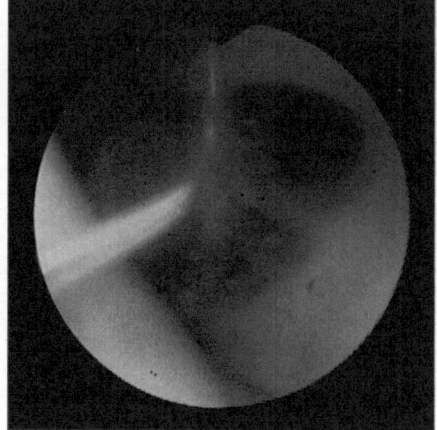

Fig. 5.93 *(left)*. Angioscopically after percutaneous thrombectomy masses of wall-adherent thrombotic material can be observed

Fig. 5.94 *(right)*. After the thrombectomy the final result shows thrombotic material on the vein wall, partially moving. The guide wire passes easily the now patent vein

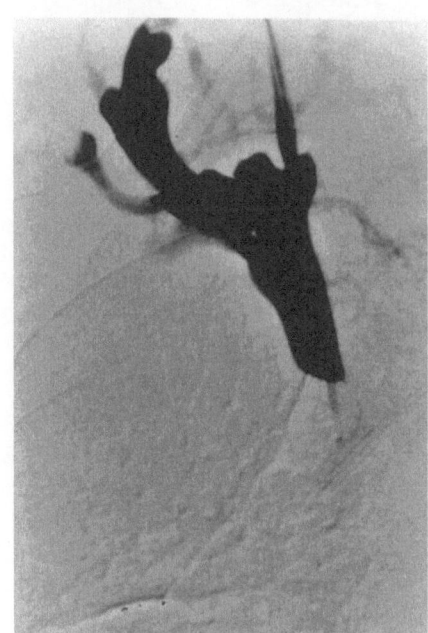

Fig. 5.95. A 50-year-old female suffering from a venous thrombosis of the right subclavian vein caused by a permanent central transjugular catheter

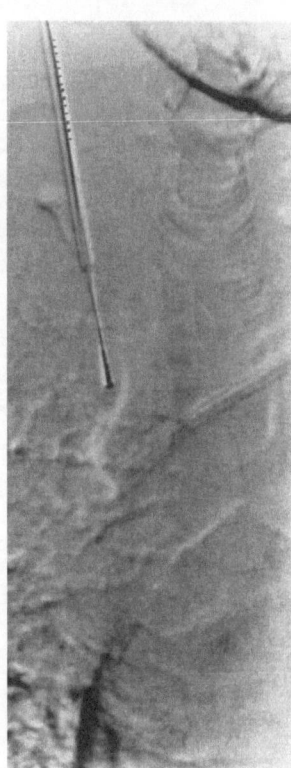

Fig. 5.96. During the thrombus extraction. The drill is positioned into the thrombus

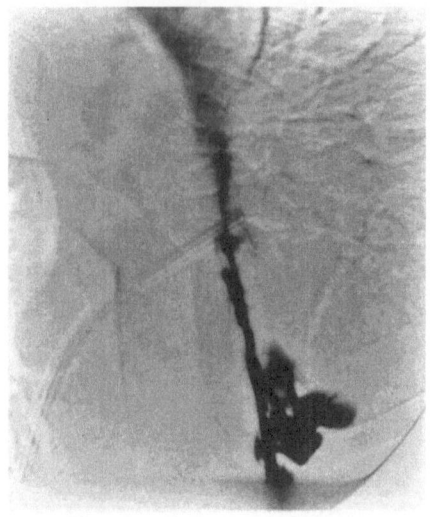

Fig. 5.97. After partial recanalization of the vein the beginning blood flow can reach the right atrium

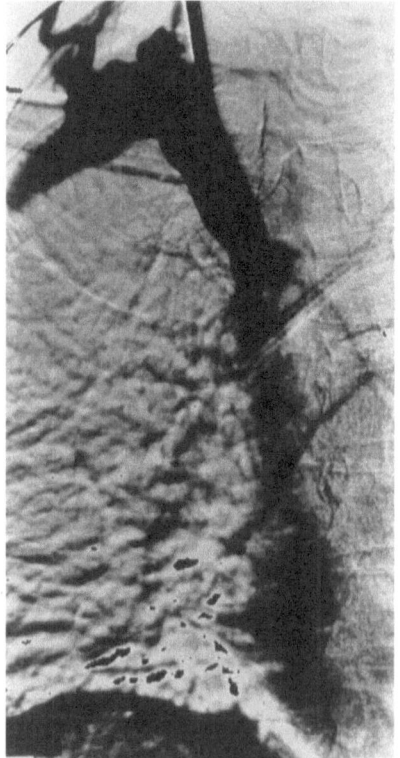

Fig. 5.98. After complete recanalization the subclavian vein is patent

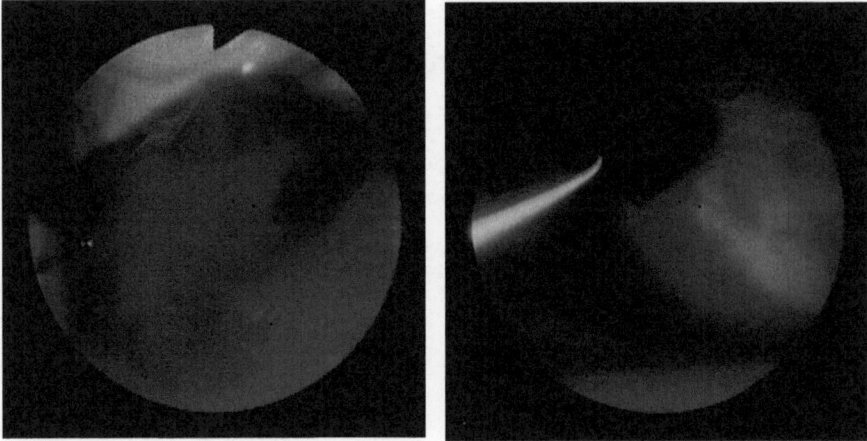

Fig. 5.99. Complete thrombotic occlusion of the subclavian vein before recanalization

Fig. 5.100. After recanalization by percutaneous thrombectomy, severe wall-adherent residual thrombi can be observed

6 Conclusions

Angiography has progressed to ever more differentiated and meticulous diagnostic procedures. The first examination of postmortem arteries in 1896 by Haschek and Lindenthal [182] was followed 27 years later by the first usable angiograms in patients by Berberich and Hirsch [69]. Interventional angiography developed over a period of 10 years from the first vascular dilatation by Dotter and Judkins [126–130] to the introduction of various angiographic methods, such as embolization [164], mechanical thrombus extraction [14, 36, 47, 55, 64], laser therapy [1–6, 24–26], and stent implantation [65, 123, 145, 297–299, 353].

PTA is a new method which has not yet found broad application because of numerous technical and mechanical problems. Reduction in the diameter of optical fibers to less than 1 mm was technically impossible for a long time. The interest of interventional radiologists especially at Freiburg University Hospital in obtaining better insight than by angiography alone into the mechanism of dilatation, local thrombolysis, and other percutaneous therapeutic methods led finally to the production of the first angioscopic prototypes [40, 115]. Several technical problems make the use of PTA difficult on a routine basis. The currently available fiberoptic angioscopes have a diameter of 0.7–2.4 mm, and the handling can therefore differ from that of endoscopes used in gastroenterology. The inadvertently intra- or extracorporal bending of the angioscope or the advancement against a resistance within the introducer sheath or the vascular lumen causes damage to optical fibers so that extensive experience with this technique is mandatory before practical use in vivo. The entire equipment must be examined before each endoscopic procedure to prevent unnecessary difficulties during the procedure. The introducer sheaths must be tested for size because the optical tip of the endoscopes can vary up to 0.4 mm in diameter. In our view, the guide wires must be tested to ensure that they pass through the biopsy channel, because of size variations in the equipment which make angioscopy impossible.

Advancing the angioscope against resistance in the introducer sheath or the vessel can damage or even destroy the highly vulnerable optical tip of the endoscope. A prerequisite for intravascular angioscopy and for the prevention of complications is the skilled and precise handling of the angiographic equipment, using the Seldinger technique. Turning the guide wire or catheter is a standard procedure in angiography for selective probing of vessels or passing stenoses. This is strictly prohibited in angioscopy as optical fibers can easily be damaged. If situations arise requiring the angioscope to be turned, it must be pulled back completely and a larger selective catheter introduced. The endoscope can be advanced again through the catheter to the region of interest. This procedure demands a skilled and experienced interventional radiologist. In our view, this procedure of "endoscopy within an angiographic catheter" has made examination of central vascular regions such as the renal arteries or supra-aortic branches possible without previously blocking the vascular lumen by a wedge catheter.

An additional technical problem in angioscopy is achieving a bloodless field within the vessel. Using an ipsilateral or contralateral balloon catheter prolongs the procedure unnecessarily and causes increased stress to the patient. When angioscopy is performed in an antegrade manner through the femoral artery, the technique of manual compression above the inguinal ligament by an assistant has been shown to be the most favorable. This is the safest and most effective way, since the blood flow is only reduced for a short time. This problem of short-term removal of blood from the vessel has been reported by other groups [42, 45, 57, 74, 99, 106, 137, 138, 146, 158], and at present it makes angioscopy technically too difficult for routine diagnostic use. The lumen of the biopsy channel is too small for flushing with a large amount of sodium chloride solution. The diameter of the angioscopes that we use is 0.7–1.9 mm. This size allows adequate sodium chloride flushing through the biopsy channel. When angioscopes with a diameter of more than 2 mm are used, larger introducer sheaths and guide catheters must also be introduced. The use of these sizes is prohibited in routine angiography because of their high rate of complications [141, 151, 157, 327]. The situation is different in the coronary arteries, according to Chaux et al. [99], Lee et al. [247, 248], Spears et al. [348–350], and Tanabe et al. [356], since only small-diameter angioscopes without biopsy channels are used as the sodium chloride solution is flushed through the large diagnostic coronary catheters.

In our experience, angioscopes with a diameter of less than 1.5 mm have major deficiencies in view of the light emission in the region observed because of the size of angioscope and the necessity to reduce the number of light fibers. The optical fibers are not reduced because the quality of the picture must not be influenced. When the vessel diameter is greater than 1.4 cm, the diameter of the endoscope must be at least 1.4 mm to enable adequate evaluation of the vessel. A smaller angioscope limits visualization only of parts of the vessel.

The results of angioscopic imaging should be recorded by continuous videotaping. Photography using an automatic winder camera usually yields inadequate results because of slow adjustment of the exposure meter.

In 1985 Ferris et al. [137, 138] reported on the first experiments of PTA in the peripheral veins of a dog. Later Mehigan [275, 276] was the first to introduce the recording on videotape in coronary angioscopy. This opened the way for angioscopy as an alternative to intraoperative coronary angiography.

Most of the angioscopic procedures reported since have used surgical access with surgical ligation of the vessel. These procedures have the advantage of no time limitation, in contrast to the percutaneous approach [91, 137, 356]. The quality of these endoscopic images of vessels totally free of blood is much better than that of images made using a short angioscopic sodium chloride flush. The problem of high-quality angioscopic recording has been overcome by forced sodium chloride flush performed in the manner described above.

The quality of the angioscopic recording depends on several factors, not only on the quality of the endoscopic optical system. This is supported by the fact that the results of other research groups have demonstrated angioscopic images of mostly inferior quality using similar or even identical angioscopic equipment [20, 59, 364–366, 368, 397]. The experience of the operator is probably the most important factor in obtaining good angioscopic results, especially with a brief blood reduction and forced sodium chloride flush.

Another important cause of varying image picture quality from the different research groups is the variety of photographic and videorecording equipment being used. The camera with a motor winder used initially by us is only partially appropriate for documentation, as about 50% of the photographs taken do not fulfill quality standards. A uniform photographic exposure is impossible since, for example, arteriosclerosis and thrombosis differ completely in color and therefore require different exposure times. On the other hand, the adjustment of a variable diaphragm using a fixed exposure time is not fast enough either because of a rapidly changing object or the rapid passage of blood and perfusing solution mixture. This may lead to loss of quality. A videocamera, however, allows dynamic recording, although single images from videotapes do not meet the quality needed for accurate diagnosis, as Fleisher et al. [140], Olcott [294], Sanborn et al. [320, 321], and Spears et al. [350] have reported.

The cold light source does not usually cause problems or complications in gastroscopic procedures, but it may be a problem in PTA. In endoscopy of the gastroenterological tract the power of the light source once adjusted to the sensitivity of the film and the exposure time is maintained throughout the procedure, whereas this method is applicable in only very few cases in angioscopy. Poor quality of the angioscopic images is probably caused by over- or underexposure of the film. Higher light power is mandatory for local thrombosis, with a red to black color spectrum, than that for atherosclerotic vessels, being predominantly white or gray in color.

The technique of sodium chloride perfusion described in this volume is similar to that used by Cortis et al. [106], Litvack et al. [255–258], Rizk et al. [316], and Towne and Bernhard [363, 364], although these other groups used smaller volumes of physiological sodium chloride solution and a lower perfusion pressure. These are important reasons for the diminished quality of their angioscopic recordings. Perfusion with sodium chloride has not led to any complications in our patients. In general, the sodium chloride perfusion should be limited to 250 ml per angioscopy and should be reduced by 50% in patients with cardiac failure. The endoscope must be positioned under X-ray control, and currently this remains the only way of controlling the angioscopic procedure. This view is in accord with the reports of Greenstone et al. [169], Raso et al. [310], Spears et al. [348–350], and Towne and Bernhardt [363, 364]. PTA with the currently available equipment and X-ray control has shown itself to be time saving and safe for the patient. Up to now no dissenting reports have been published. Only in intraoperative examination of vascular anastomoses can X-ray control be omitted [348, 349].

The complications of X-ray control during angioscopy do not differ from those during angiography, as the diameter of the endoscope is similar to the angiographic catheter sizes. Only the tip of the angioscope is larger than the catheter tip. Therefore the angioscope must be used with care when advanced in the vessel so as to prevent vascular dissections and embolization of mural thrombotic material. According to our data and the observations of other groups, forced sodium chloride flush has not caused any complications so far [321]. Problems may perhaps be caused by sterilization temperatures exceeding 50°C, which may damage the angioscopic optical system. We sterilize our angioscopes in the same way as Sanborn et al. [320, 321] and Towne and Bernhardt [363, 364]. Neither these authors nor we have observed any infection related to the angioscopic procedure.

Angioscopic procedures in patients are still limited to central and peripheral vessels greater than 1.5 mm in diameter. Besides the diameter of the angioscope, the size of the channel is also important for angioscopic imaging since this is crucial for adequate sodium chloride flushing. One solution to this problem is the occlusion of the proximal vessel by a wedge balloon catheter positioned right in front of the tip of the angioscope. We have not used this method so far as vascular occlusion must be achieved before each angioscopic view, and simple inflation of a balloon catheter for vascular occlusion might injure the intima. In our opinion, the additional risk of this procedure is not justifiable.

Angioscopy reveals several findings which are usually diagnosed only by pathological examination. The differentiation between local thrombosis and thromboembolism is not ascertained by angiography. This is in accordance with findings of Auster et al. [27], Dotter and Judkins [127, 128], Fischer [139], and Katzen et al. [226, 227]. Also, the accurate grading of the severity of atherosclerosis is not possible, a problem that may lead to false measurement and subsequent treatment [232, 243, 408]. Likewise, severe vascular stenoses caused by multiple plaques are of major importance for the indication of angioplasty. In the cerebral arteries angioscopy can be essential in deciding whether to perform angioplasty because it enables direct examination of the stenosis. Inflammatory and actinic vascular injuries can be diagnosed, and diagnosis of these lesions has previously been achieved by histological examination [41, 180].

In addition to Block's classification of atherosclerosis based on anatomical and pathological findings [77–79], angioscopy can establish the prognosis and possible therapeutic action for the patient. This is in addition to diagnosing vascular stenosis, partial thrombosis, or atherosclerotic plaques, findings that are in agreement with reports of Chaux et al. [99], Cortis et al. [106], Grundfest et al. [175–179], and Sanborn [321]. Angiographically diagnosed stenoses can be subdivided by angioscopy into lipoidosis, sclerosis, atheroma, inflammatory granulating tissue, and thrombosis. In contrast, angiography is superior to angioscopy in examining tiny vessels and in evaluating the parenchymal and venous phases of the vascular system.

Pathological vascular changes such as inflammatory, actinic, and early atherosclerotic lesions are diagnosed at an earlier stage by angioscopy than by angiography. This has been confirmed by the observations of Guthaner and Schmitz in 1982 [180]. Obscure vascular stenoses in young patients without systemic illnesses can often not be classified by angiography [63, 155, 373]. Angiographic criteria of inflammatory vascular diseases are only discrete, and, according to Voigt and Goerttler [381], Hasso et al. [185], and Guthaner and Schmitz [180], unequivocal diagnosis is sometimes impossible. However, the diagnosis of inflammatory vascular disease can be made without any difficulty by angioscopy. Actinic vascular injury remains the only differential diagnosis.

In introducing interventional, angioscopically controlled dilatation, recanalization, and local lysis, we have entered new angiographic ground; earlier this was only performed in coronary arteries by Chaux et al. [99], Lee et al. [247], Mehigan [276], Spears et al. [348–350], and Tanabe et al. (356].

Several hypotheses have been established for the pathological-morpho-logical mechanism of balloon dilatation and vascular recanalization. Grünt-zig's [172, 173] theory of atherosclerotic plaque compression by angioplasty has recently been opposed by Block et al. [77–79], Castaneda-Zuniga et al. [97], Kinney et al. [232], Laerum et al. [243], and Wolf et al. [408]. These authors have histologically observed dissections of the intima and media after dilatation of the atherosclerotic plaque [97]. A deformation of the prominent parts of the atherosclerotic plaque is observed angioscopically after angio-plasty. However, this adds little to the enlargement of the vascular lumen. The histological findings of Wolf et al. [408], Zollikofer et al. [419–421], Kinney et al. [232], and Castaneda-Zuniga et al. [97] that angioplasty causes intimal dissection with primarily longitudinal tears through the plaque have been confirmed by in vivo angioscopy. The instability of the arterial wall after angioplasty in the presence of an eccentric residual lumen has been visualized by angioscopy. The angiographic findings of immediate restenosis after technically successful angioplasty can be explained by these mechanisms. Gardiner et al. [157], Martin et al. [267], Motarjeme et al. [285], and Lamerton [245] have reported occasional complete vascular occlusions after PTA. It must be assumed that vascular instability is the reason for their observations. The lumen cannot be kept open because of a reduction in blood pressure caused by additional proximal stenosis of the vessel.

Tears of atheromatous plaques with successive mural thrombosis after vascular dilatation are the main reason for high early reocclusion rates after angioplasty, and this has been shown as a direct cause by angioscopy. The longer the tears of the atheromatous plaques the higher is the probability of restenosis or thrombotic vascular occlusion. The hypothesis that dilatation of the vessel above the normal size is necessary for good results is no longer justifiable in the light of our angioscopic findings [154, 172, 240]. Angioplastic dilatation above the normal vascular cross-sectional size may lead to an immediate angiographic success if the vascular stability is maintained, although it has a higher risk of thrombosis in the long term, especially when anticoagulation is not continued.

Complications in vascular segments distal to the dilated segment have been reported after balloon dilatation by Schrempp et al. [327], Simonetti et al. [341], and Weibull et al. [388]. Causes of these complications can be evaluated by angioscopy. The observations of Anderson et al. [19], Lamerton [245], and Castaneda-Zuniga et al. [97] that protruding atheromatous plaques cannot break off during balloon catheterization must be questioned. Parts of plaques can embolize to the periphery where they are obviously insoluble to local lysis. Wall-adherent thrombi have also been shown to be susceptible to embolization when loosened by guide wires or catheter dilatation.

Inflammatory and actinic vascular injuries have been treated with angioplasty [41, 180] in only few patients so that little experience is currently available. Angioscopic comparisons have not been reported so far. The elasticity of the vessels is irrelevantly reduced in both conditions so that these stenoses cannot be completely dilated.

The procedure of local lysis was introduced 20 years ago and has been modified and evaluated by angioscopy. Angioscopy can differentiate very well between local thrombosis and embolism and thereby influence therapeutic procedures. An extended embolus would not be tested with local catheter lysis but would be considered for surgical intervention or thrombus extraction. Administering the thrombolytic material through the angioscope has the advantage of immediate control of the thrombolytic results. In addition, angioscopy has the advantage of determining the prognosis by evaluating the vascular state directly after thrombolysis. There is no reduction in radiation time with angioscopy, in contrast to angiography, since angioscopy requires X-ray control.

Recently, vascular prostheses have increasingly been recognized as a therapeutic procedure, although Dotter and colleagues had already invented and used the first model in animals in 1983 [126]. The present stents have been positioned either by surgical access with catheters [127] or by PTA technique [45, 50, 132, 272, 297–299, 353]. In 1986 Palmaz and coworkers [297] reported on an extendable intraluminal vascular prosthesis that was implanted into the vessel using a 12-F introducer sheath. In 1969, Dotter [127] described a coil that expanded after the guide wire had been removed from the stent. Cragg and coworkers [108, 109] also reported on a nitinol prosthesis in 1984, the shape of which was sensitive to heat; it was maintained in a compressed shape by the cold but returned to its original larger shape at body temperature, thus keeping the vascular lumen open. These stents have been implanted only in animals, and several differing results have been reported. Only recent studies by Strecker et al. [353] and Palmaz et al. [297, 298] have reported on large numbers of patients treated by stent implantation. Palmaz et al. [299] have reported that two out of six endoprostheses showed recurrent stenosis because of new and severe intimal hyperplasia. In animals which were not heparinized two partial and one complete occlusions have been observed.

In our animal studies we avoided using heparin to be able angioscopically to follow thrombosis occurring as a direct result of stent implantation. A thrombotic occlusion of stents has not been observed so far, which indicates a low thrombotic potential of the endoprosthetic material. We are currently awaiting long-term follow-up results and histological analysis. In our opinion, angioscopy is the method of choice for evaluating endoprostheses; this provides information regarding function, degree of stenosis, thrombogeneity, and the neointimal reaction. Histological analysis of vessels from animals cannot satisfactorily answer all the questions of stent implantation. In particular the development of a new intima on the inside of the stent within 2–3 months [299] has an impact on prognosis and supports the necessity of intraluminal stent examination. Angiography is able to detect the degree of restenosis or thrombosis, but it is certainly inferior to angioscopy in evaluating the intimal lining of the stent.

The stent construction of gilded brass lattice with worked-in silver reinforcements has proven very satisfactory in our experiments. No stent showed evidence of breakage, bending, or other changes of the material suggestive of wear. An analysis of the histological changes induced by stent implantation has not yet been possible because of excellent results in animal studies as well as patients. Currently, angioscopic reports of intraluminal stents have not yet been published.

Vascular endoprostheses are an alternative to surgical bypass of vascular occlusions in the distal femoral and popliteal arteries. Studies on the late results of PTA point to the problem of worse long-term results in distal vascular segments with a high incidence of reocclusions, as reported by Lu, Probst, Wierny, and their coworkers [261, 306, 406]. Therefore a vascular prosthesis seems sensible in these distal segments to maintain "permanent dilatation." In the pelvic region, particularly near the bifurcation, a similar procedure is conceivable. In our opinion, a stent implantation in the pelvic region should be considered only when the possibility of successful conventional PTA therapy has been exhausted because conventional balloon dilatation has been shown to have the best early and late results in this region [46, 50, 65].

Implantation of stents in the trifurcational region of the lower limb, the popliteal or the renal artery will be important in the future. In these regions preceding angioscopic examination will probably become more accepted and used in the future. Stents will have to be improved in stability and flexibility especially for use in regions of joint bending.

In our view, implantation of vascular prostheses into vessels, especially in the pelvic region or femoral and popliteal arteries that have previously been dilated, is certainly worth trying prior to bypass surgery. In addition, implantation of endoprostheses into severely eccentric stenoses of the iliac arteries is advancing and has already been clinically tested in 30 patients at Freiburg University Hospital using the method of Palmaz et al. [297–299]. The results are encouraging. The implantation of one stent into the distal popliteal region proximal to the trifurcation has been performed successfully by our group [45]. One major problem still remaining is metal fatigue and thus the danger of breakage. In view of this, other materials such as plastic may have to be considered.

Percutaneous transluminal thrombus extraction in the manner described, with simultaneous angioscopic control, is novel. Current interventional radiological techniques for restoring blood flow after vascular thrombosis include the angioplastic techniques of Dotter and Judkins [128] and Grüntzig [172, 173], the local lysis procedures of Hess et al. [189–191] and Totty et al. [362], the laser therapy of Choy et al. [102], Geschwind et al. [159, 160], Abela et al. [1–11], and Ashworth et al. [26], thrombus extraction techniques similar to the Fogarty thrombus extraction, and the percutaneous thrombus extraction with a catheter system by Buxton and Mueller [92], Sniderman et al. [346], and Starck et al. [351]. One aim of our work has been to establish a novel method that can be used without risk in addition to angioplasty for the extraction of fresh or old thrombotic material. An angioscopic control of this procedure in addition to conventional angiography seems mandatory as definitive results of the intravascular condition after thrombus extraction are still lacking. A clinical use of percutaneous thrombus extraction, on the other hand, is indicated, and alternative procedures have been developed since encouraging long-term results with local catheter lysis are rare.

Other groups have reported the results of thrombus extraction by different catheter systems that have been used with only partial success [346, 351]. It seems sensible to use percutaneous thrombectomy in combination with local lysis if thrombolysis is incomplete. On the other hand, it is also possible mechanically to clear most of the thrombotic material first and thereby reduce the dose of the thrombolytic agent. Our method seems appropriate for use in vascular regions below the inguinal ligament. Within the inguinal region Fogarty's procedure [141] is the established technique because of the good clinical results. Fogarty's procedure requires surgical access which is generally not available for the interventional radiologist. Since the introduction of this method in 1963 it has been shown to be relatively free of complications in comparison with other techniques [318]. Distal to the inguinal ligament the Fogarty method seems inferior to percutaneous thrombus extraction because it lacks angiographic or angioscopic control. Dissections in peripheral vascular regions can therefore not be detected. In addition to possible dissections, the method of Fogarty has the disadvantage of loosening thrombotic material with consequent peripheral embolism and occlusion of the collateral vessels by the balloon catheter. Percutaneous thrombus extraction, on the other hand, is based on the principle of negative pressure at the catheter tip, with constant suction of thrombotic material into the catheter and simultaneous cutting of· the thrombus into fragments. Thromboembolism using this technique is less likely.

Percutaneous thrombectomy has the additional advantage of being able to extract thrombotic material distal to the femoral artery. The frequency of complications of percutaneous thrombus extraction probably does not exceed that of local lysis or balloon dilatation. Because of the small number of cases, direct comparison between the different therapeutic techniques is currently not possible. Considering the technical procedure, an additional risk compared to PTA or local lysis cannot be expected. Several long-term follow-up studies of PTA have shown a total rate of complications of about 4% and a mortality rate below 0.1% [50, 57, 306, 318]. These rates will not be increased by the introduction of thrombus extraction, but will probably be lower because of the limitation in number of local catheter thrombolyses. For successful percutaneous thrombus extraction the radiologist must have extensive experience with conventional methods of PTA and local thrombolysis.

Angioscopy is an ideal method for the control of interventional procedures. The direct vision of thrombus extraction by angioscopy has been performed only in animal studies as two different catheter accesses for thrombus extraction catheter and angioscopy must be simultaneously used. If smaller sizes of endoscopes and thrombus extraction devices are developed, the angioscope and the thrombus extraction device could be introduced through one introducer sheath. The possibility of thrombus extraction under direct sight could revolutionize therapeutic decision making for local lysis of the residual thrombotic material, dilatation, conservative management, and vascular surgery.

As an additional method, percutaneous thrombus extraction seems to be a sensible and important aid for the therapeutic management of thrombosis that can effectively support local lysis and partially even replace it. Within the spectrum of diagnostic and interventional methods of vascular disease percutaneous transluminal angioscopy has initiated a new era. Endoscopy of the gastrointestinal tract has been firmly established in diagnosis since its first use 20 years ago. Is it possible that angioscopy is a similar boon? Because of the highly technical and time-consuming nature of percutaneous transluminal angioscopy this method will be used in the near future only for single problems that cannot be solved by the established angiological methods. In the fields of stent implantation, control of rotation angioplasty, thrombus extraction, and laser angioplasty, angioscopy has already become an important diagnostic tool for precise control of vascular procedures under direct vision.

Many questions about the mechanism of these interventional procedures and their impact on the vascular system, such as the discussions about the mechanism of angioplasty from Grüntzig [172, 173] to Zollikofer et al. [419–421], may be answered in advance by angioscopy.

A major influence on the number of angiographic procedures similar to the decline of radiological examinations by endoscopy of the gastrointestinal tract is not expected. Even with the technical improvement of angioscopy this method will be dependent on concomitant radiological examination. Nevertheless, percutaneous angioscopy is an additional and definitely promising new method that will eventually be integrated into the spectrum of routine angiographic examination procedures.

7 Future Aspects of Percutaneous Angioscopy

With the development of angioscopes less than 2 mm in diameter, it has become possible to examine the vascular system by percutaneous transluminal angioscopy and to visualize regions of human arteries previously visualized only by angiography. A necessity for the introduction of this method was the occlusion of blood flow in the vascular region of interest. This has been solved and clinically tested by a technically simple method.

Angioscopy permits the differentiation between local thrombosis and thromboembolism and allows precise evaluation of atherosclerosis and actinic vascular changes. Furthermore, angiographic stenoses can be distinguished angioscopically as lipoidosis, sclerosis, atheroma, inflammation, or new or old thrombosis.

For the first time interventional procedures such as dilatation, recanalization, and local thrombolysis could be directly controlled and visualized by angioscopy. The mechanism of balloon dilatation was demonstrated in vivo, thereby providing new insight into the pathophysiological mechanisms. The frequent recurrent vascular occlusions after balloon dilatation were shown to be due mostly to an arterial wall instability induced by angioplasty.

Local catheter thrombolysis has been continuously monitored by angioscopy. Embolization of thrombotic material has been observed during catheter lysis. Additionally, peripheral embolization of atherosclerotic plaques or mural thrombi have been observed angioscopically during the introduction of guide wires and catheters.

The development of a new vascular endoprosthesis has shown encouraging clinical results. For the first time it has been possible to perform controlled examinations under direct vision and to evaluate the new intimal lining of stents by angioscopy. A new device for percutaneous transluminal thrombus extraction has been established as an alternative method for the high-risk local catheter thrombolysis. The thrombus extraction device and the vascular endoprosthesis are certainly novel and exciting instruments for the interventional radiologist.

Overall, percutaneous transluminal angioscopy has its place within the field of percutaneous diagnostic and interventional methods. Although angioscopy is currently not used on a routine basis, it is nonetheless of great help in difficult interventional procedures and is capable of answering specific questions that are not resolved by other diagnostic methods.

References

1. Abela G, Norman S, Cohen D, Feldman R, Geiser F, Conti C (1982) Effects of carbon dioxide, Nd-YAG and argon laser radiation on coronary atheromatous plaques. Am J Cardiol 50: 1199–1205
2. Abela G, Normann S, Cohen D (1985) Laser recanalization of occluded atherosclerotic arteries in vivo and in vito. Circulation 71: 403
3. Abela G, Staples E, Conti C, Pepine C,Varo R, Knauf D, Alexander J, Hey D, Roberts A (1983) Immediate and long term effects of laser radiation on the arterial wall: light and electron microscopic observation. Surg Forum 3: 454–456
4. Abela G, Seeger J, Khoury A, Jablonski S, Conti R (1988) Peripheral artery laser recanalization. J Am Coll Cardiol 11 (2): 107A
5. Abela G (1988) Laser arterial recanalization: a current perspective. J Am Coll Cardiol 12 (1): 103–105
6. Abela G, Seeger J, Khoury A, Jablonski S, Conti C (1987) Laser recanalization of peripheral arteries in humans: acute and long term effects. Circulation 76 [Suppl IV]: 409
7. Abela G, Fenech A, Crea F, Conti C (1985) Hot tip: another method of laser vascular recanalization. Lasers Surg Med 5: 327–335
8. Abela G, Orea F, Seeger J (1985) The healing process in normal canine arteries and in atherosclerotic monkey arteries after transluminal laser irradiation. Am J Cardiol 56: 983–988
9. Abela G, Seeger J, Barbieri E, Franzini D, Fenech A, Pepine C, Conti C (1986) Laser angioplasty with angioscopic guidance in humans. J Am Coll Cardiol 8: 184–192
10. Abela G, Crea F, Smith W, Pepine C, Conti C (1985) In vitro effects of argon laser radiation on blood: quantitative and morphologic analysis. J Am Coll Cardiol 5: 231–237
11. Abela G,Tomaru T, Mansour M, Barbeau G, Kaelin L, Seeger J, Caravallo J (1990) Reduced platelet deposition with laser compared to balloon angioplasty. J Am Coll Cardiol 15 (2): 245A
12. Abrams HL, Adams DF (1969) The coronary arteriogram. N Engl J Med 281: 1276–1285
13. Adcock O, Adcock G,Wheeler J (1984) Optimal techniques for harvesting preparation of reversed autogenous vein grafts for use as arterial substitutes: a review. Surgery 96: 886–893
14. Ahn S, Auth D, Marcus D, Moore W (1988) Removal of focal atheromatous lesions by angioscopically guided high-speed rotary atherectomy: preliminary experimental observations. J Vasc Surg 7: 292–300
15. Alken CE, Sommer F (1950) Die Renovasographie. Z Urol 43: 420
16. Allen D, Graham E (1922) Intracardiac surgery – a new method. J Am Med Assoc 79: 1028–1030
17. Allen D (1924) Intracardiac surgery. AMA Arch Surg 8: 317–319
18. Almagor Y, Leon M, Bartorelli A, Lenhard S, Perlman M, Follmann D, Roberts W (1989) Media thinning of severely diseased coronary arteries: guidelines for new interventional procedures. J Am Coll Cardiol 13 (2): 194A

104   References

19. Anderson C, Collins G, Pich N (1978) Routine operative arteriography during carotid endarterectomy: a reassessment. Surgery 83: 67–71
20. Anderson H, Zaatari G, Roubin C, Leimsgruber P, Gruentzig A (1986) Steerable fiber optic catheter delivery of laser energy in atherosclerotic rabbits. Am Heart J 111: 1065–1072
21. Anderson JB, Wolinski HP, Wels IP, Willins DC, Bliss BP (1986) The impact of PTA on the management of peripheral vascular disease. Br J Surg 73: 17–18
22. Anger P, Wenz W (1981) Aus der Pionierzeit der Arteriographie. Radiologie 21: 65–71
23. Anon J (1987) Looking inside arteries. Lancet 2: 374–375
24. Ascher P, Lammer G, Choy D (1987) Eradication of carotid artery obstruction with the argon laser. Lasers 3: 25–29
25. Ashley S, Gehani A, Brooks S, Davies A, Ball S, Rees M (1988) The use of angioscopy in experimental laser and dynamic angioplasty. Heart Vessels 4: 49
26. Ashworth E, Dalsinf M, Olson J, Baughman S, Reuilly M, Glover J (1987) Laser assisted vascular anastomoses of larger arteries. Lasers 3: 33–39
27. Auster M, Kadir S, Mitchel SE, Williams GM, Perler BA, Chang R, Whithe RI Jr (1984) Iliac artery occlusion: management with intrathrombus streptokinase infusion and angioplasty. Radiology 153: 385
28. Axon A, Phillips I, Cotton P, Avery S (1974) Disinfection of gastrointestinal fibre endoscopes. Lancet 1: 656–658
29. Balko A, Piasecki C, Shah D, Carney W, Hopkins R, Jackson B (1986) Transfemoral placement of intraluminal polyurethane prosthesis for abdominal aortic aneurysm. J Surg Res 40: 305–309
30. Bandyk D, Kaebnick H, Stewart G, Towne J (1987) Durability of the in-situ saphenous vein arterial bypass: a comparison of primary and secondary patency. J Vasc Surg 5: 256–268
31. Barath P, Litvack F, Grundfest W, Forrester J (1988) Combined angioplasty and vascular stenting by a novel heat-expandable thermoplastic device. J Am Coll Cardiol 11 (2): 65A
32. Bar-Meir S, Rotmensch S (1987) A comparison between peroral choledochoscopy and endoscopic retrograde cholangiopancreaticography. Gastrointest Endosc 33: 13–19
33. Barth KH (1983) Modified catheter for transluminal angioplasty of the femoropopliteal artery. Radiology 149: 598–599
34. Bartorelli A, Potkin B, Almagor Y, Gessert J, Roberts W, Leon M (1989) Intravascular ultrasound imaging of atherosclerotic coronary arteries: an in vitro validation study. J Am Coll Cardiol 13 (2): 4A
35. Bartorelli A, Bonner R, Almagor Y, Neville R, Mcintosh C, Swain J, Leon M (1989) Enhanced recognition of plaque composition in vivo using laser-excited fluorescence spectroscopy. J Am Coll Cardiol 13 (2): 54A
36. Battler A, Scheinowitz M, Rath S, Boseck C, Eldar M (1989) Bard rotary atherectomy system (BRAS) in normal canine coronary arteries. J Am Coll Cardiol 13 (2): 223A
37. Bauriedel C, Höfling B (1988) Adjunctive angioscopy during percutaneous atherectomy. Eur Heart J 9 [Suppl A]: 123
38. Bauriedel G, von Pölnitz A, Simpson J, Höfling B (1989) Angioskopie bei Gefäßverschlüssen und perkutaner Rekanalisation. Z Kardiol 78 [Suppl I]: 106
39. Beatt K, Bertrand M, Puel J, Rickards T, Serruys P, Sigwart U (1989) Additional improvement in vessel lumen in the first 24 hours after stent implantation due to radial dilating force. J Am Coll Cardiol 13 (2): 224A
40. Beck A (1987) Perkutane Angioskopie: erste Erfahrungsberichte der PTA und der lokalen Lyse unter angioskopischen Bedingungen. Radiologe 27: 555–559
41. Beck A, Eble M, Huber K (1989) Angioskopie der aktinisch geschädigten A. subclavia vor und nach Angioplastie. CV World Report 2 (3): 101–106

42. Beck A, Grosser G, Hellwig A, Papacharalampous X (1987) Ultraschallkontrolle der Katheterdilatation. In: Hansmann M, Koischwitz D, Lutz H, Trier H (eds) Ultraschalldiagnostik 1986. Springer Berlin Heidelberg New York, 190–192

43. Beck A, Grosser G, Hellwig A, Papacharalampous X (1987) Ultraschallgesteuerte Kontrolle der lokalen Lyse. In: Hansmann M, Koischwitz D, Lutz H, Trier H (eds) Ultraschalldiagnostik 1986. Springer, Berlin Heidelberg New York, 193–195

44. Beck A, Ott D (1988) Percutaneous transluminal angioscopy of supraaortic branches and angioscopical control of PTA. In: Nadjimi M (ed) Imaging of brain metabolism, spine and cord, interventional radiology. Springer, Berlin Heidelberg New York, pp 329–333

45. Beck A, Nanko N (1988) Angioskopische Kontrolle der perkutanen Gefäßendoprothese – Erfahrungsbericht über ein speziell entwickeltes transfemorales Gefäßendoprothesenmodell und dessen angioskopische Kontrolle in situ. Cor Vasa 3: 119–123

46. Beck A, Ostheim-Dzerowycz W, Grosser G, Heiss HW (1988) Klinische und angiographische Langzeitergebnisse der perkutanen transluminalen Angioplastie und der lokalen Katheterlyse der supraaortalen Becken- und Beingefäße. Cor Vasa 2: 1022–1034

47. Beck A, Reinbold WD, Blum U, Nanko N, Milic S, Papacharalampous X (1988) Clinical application of percutaneous transluminal angioscopy. Comparison of findings in percutaneous transluminal angioplasty, thrombolysis, thrombus-extraction and stent application. Herz: 392–399

48. Beck A, Eble M, Huber K (1989) Angioskopie der aktinisch geschädigten A. subclavia vor und nach Angioplastie. CV World Report 2: 101–106

49. Beck A, Blum U (1989) Die Angioskopie der perkutanen transluminalen Angioplastie (PTA) von Subclaviastenosen. Cor Vasa 3: 87–91

50. Beck A, Egheoni C, Milic S, Spagnoli AM (1989) The long term effects of percutaneous transluminal angioplasty, local catheter lysis and stent-implantation. Clin Ter 131: 149–164

51. Beck A, Milic S, Dinkel E, Blum U, Papacharalampous X (1989) Arterielle Gefäßendoskopie und lokale Lysetherapie. CV World Report 2: 190–195

52. Beck A, Milic S, Friedburg H, Mundinger A, Licht T, Spagnoli AM, Egheoni C (1989) The value of percutaneous cholangioscopy and stent implantation in inoperable carcinoma of the bile-duct using a new endoprothesis. Prog Rep 1: 95–106

53. Beck A, Milic S, Spagnoli AM, Mundinger A, Blum U (1989) The clinical value of percutaneous transluminal angioscopy: angioscopical findings in primary vascular diagnosis and in interventional radiology. Clin Ter 131: 93–105

54. Beck A, Milic S (1989) Dilatation of the carotid artery by a temporary carotid filter – first results of percutaneous transluminal angioscopy. Oplitai 2: 123–129

55. Beck A, Hauenstein KH, Blum U, Nanko N, Milic S (1989) Percutaneous transluminal angioscopy: comparison of findings in percutaneous transluminal angioplasty, thrombus-extraction and stent application. In: Zeitler E, Seyferth W (eds) Pros and cons in PTA and auxiliary methods. Springer, Berlin Heidelberg New York, pp 199–209

56. Beck A, Heiß H, Schmid K, Wandl J (1989) Über die perkutane transluminale Angioskopie der Aorta. Cor Vasa 6: 188–193

57. Beck A, Muhe A, Ostheim W, Heiss W, Hasler K (1989) Long-term results of percutaneous transluminal angioplasty: a study of 4750 dilatations and local lyses. Eur J Vasc Surg 3: 245–252

58. Beck A, Hauenstein KH, Salm R, Rückauer K, Nanko N, Milic S, Papacharalampous X (1989) Percutaneous transluminal angioscopy versus conventional and digital angiography: comparison of findings in percutaneous transluminal angioplasty, thrombolysis, thrombus-extraction and stent-application. In: Richter K (ed) Digitale und interventionelle Radiologie bei Herz- und Gefäßkrankheiten. Akademie, Berlin, pp 285–301

59. Beck A, Nanko N, Milic S, Volk B (1989) Stentimplantation beim inoperablen Gallengangskarzinom. Röntgenpraxis 7: 231–235

60. Beck A, Nanko N, Schildge J, Hasse J (1989) Stentimplantation als Palliativmaß-nahme beim inoperablen Bronchialtumor: erste Erfahrungen über eine endoskopisch implantierte Stentapplikation. Radiologe 8: 399–405
61. Beck A (1990) Über eine neue ballonexpandierbare Kunststoffendoprothese. Erster Erfahrungsbericht über den modellierbaren Kunststoffstent. Radiologe 30: 347–350
62. Beck A, Hauenstein KH, Volk BA, Milic S, Nanko N, Kröpelin T (1990) Percutaneous cholangioscopy and stent implantation in inoperable carcinoma of the bile duct using a new endoprothesis. Tumor Diagn Ther 2: 85–89
63. Beck A, Milic S, Spagnoli AM, Mundinger A, Nanko N, Dinkel E, Schopp D (1990) Percutaneous transluminal angioscopy: a new method for control of vascular situation. Ergeb Exp Med 52: 35–44
64. Beck A, Krause T, Mundinger A, Milic S, Papacharalampous X (1990) Über ein neues Imstrumentarium für die kathetergestützte Thrombektomie aus arteriellen und venösen Gefäßen beim Menschen – erste angioskopische Kontrollen bei der Extraktion von Lungenembolien. Ergeb Exp Med 52: 319–328
65. Beck A, Milic S, Spagnoli AM, Nanko N (1990) Kurz- und Langzeiterfahrungsbericht über ein eigenes Gefäßendoprothesenmodell und dessen angioskopische Kontrolle in situ. Ergeb Exp Med 52: 355–364
66. Beck A, Hufnagel A, Mundinger A, Vogel T, Bruker G, Stengele O (1992) Perkutane transluminale Angioskopie. Eine neue Möglichkeit zur Kontrolle der intravasalen Verhältnisse nach Dilatationen, Rekanalisationen, lokalen Lysen und Stentimplan-tationen. Kassenarzt 19: 36–44
67. Beck A, Milic St, Mundinger A, Schoop D, Spagnoli AM, Barbuto D (1992) Vascular endoscopy: current state of the art. Angioscopical and angiographical comparison in PTA, thrombolysis, thrombus extraction and stent application. Esperienze (Experi-ence) Edit Univ Rom 3: 13–29
68. Bensaude R (1956) Rectoscopie, sigmoidoscopie. Masson, Paris
69. Berberich J, Hirsch S (1923) Die röntgenographische Darstellung der Arterien und Venen am lebenden Menschen. Klin Wochenschr 49: 2226–2228
70. Berkowitz HD, Spence RK, Freimann DB, Barker CF, Roberts B, McLean G, Ring E (1983) Long term results of PTA of the femoral artery. In: Dotter CT, Grüntzig A, Schoop W, Zeitler E (eds) Percutaneous transluminal angioplasty. Springer, Berlin Heidelberg New York
71. Bernhard V (1986) Endoscopy and vascular surgery. J Vasc Surg 4: 415
72. Biamino C, Kar A, Cross M, Dörschel K, Müller C (1988) Optimization of photoablation for angioplasty using excimer laser. Eur Heart J 9 [Suppl 1]: 330
73. Biamino C, Nohla K, Skarabis P, Dörschel K, Kar N, Müller C (1989) Excimer-Laser-Guide Wire. Eine neue Technik in der Laserangioplastie. Z Kardiol 78 [Suppl 1]: 20
74. Biermann HR, Miller ER, Byron RL, Dod KS, Kelly KH, Black DH (1951) Intra-arterial catheterization of viscera in man. AJR 66: 555
75. Birnie G, Quigley E, Clements G, Follet E, Watkinson G (1983) Endoscopic transmission of hepatitis B virus. Gut 24: 171–174
76. Blaisdell F, Lim A (1967) Technical result of carotid endarterectomy arteriographic assessment. Am J Surg 114: 239–246
77. Block PC, Myler RK, Stertzer S (1982) Morphology after transluminal angioplasty in human beings. Radiology 142: 820
78. Block PC, Elmer D, Fallon JT (1983) Release of arteriosclerotic debris after transluminal angioplasty. Radiology 146: 276
79. Block W (1951) Die Durchblutungsstörungen der Gliedmaßen. de Gruyter, Berlin
80. Bockenheimer ST, Mathias K (1983) Percutaneous transluminal angioplasty in arteriosclerotic internal carotid artery stenosis. AJNR 4: 791
81. Bolton H, Bailey C, Costas-Durieux J (1954) Cardioscopy – simple and practical. J Thorac Surg 27: 323–329

82. Bonan R (1989) Percutaneous coronary angioscopy. In: Vogel J, King S (eds) Interventional cardiology: future directions. Mosby, St. Louis, pp 28–35

83. Bonan R, Bhat K, Ki Leung T, Lam J, Lemarbre L, Wolff R (1989) The self-expanding parallel wire metallic stent. J Am Coll Cardiol 13 (2): 106A

84. Bonan R, Parisella M, Fournier J, Crepeau J, Cote G, De Guise P, Waters D (1987) Percutaneous coronary angioscopy technique and results. Eur Heart J 8 [Suppl II]: 222

85. Boutin C (1989) The laser in thoracoscopy. Pneumologie 43: 96–97

86. Braun W, Lotze M, Tänzer A (1966) Vertebralisangiographie mit Hilfe des Femoraliskatheters. ROFO 104: 839–847

87. Broden B, Hanson HE, Karnell J (1948) Thoracic aortography. Acta Radiol 29: 181–186

88. Buchbinder D, Singh J, Karmody A (1981) Comparison of patency rate and structural changes of in-situ and reversed vein arterial bypass. J Surg Res 3O: 213–222

89. Buchwald A, Werner G, Unterberg C, Wiegand V (1990) Restenose nach Excimer-Laser-Angioplastie von Koronarstenosen. Z Kardiol. 79 [Suppl 1]: 21

90. Bürsch JH, Hahne HJ, Brennecke R, Heintzen PH (1983) Digitale Funktionsangiographie. Radiologe 23: 202–209

91. Butterworth R (1951) A new operating cardioscope. J Thorac Surg 22: 319–322

92. Buxton DR Jr, Mueller CF (1974) Removal of iatrogenic clot by transcatheter embolectomy. Radiology 111: 39

93. Cadranel S, Rodesch P, Cremer M (1979) Diagnostic and operative fiberendoscopy of the upper gastrointestinal tract in paediatrics. Z Kinderchir 27 [Suppl I]: 63–66

94. Carlens E (1959) Mediastinoscopy: a method for inspection and tissue biopsy in the superior mediastinum. Dis Chest 36: 343–352

95. Carlens E, Silander T (1961) Method for direct inspection of the right atrium. Experimental observation in the dog. Surgery 49: 622–624

96. Carlens E, Silander T (1963) Cardioscopy. J Cardiovasc Surg 4: 512–515

97. Castaneda-Zuniga WR, Amplatz K, Laerum F (1981) Mechanics of angioplasty: an experimental approach. Radiology 1: 1–14

98. Chandraratna P, Jones J, Rahimtoola S, Kaiser S (1989) Evaluation of mixed atherosclerotic plaques by quantitative ultrasonic methods. J Am Coll Cardiol 13 (2): SA

99. Chaux A, Lee ME, Blanche C, Kass RM, Sherman TC (1986) Intraoperative coronary angioscopy. J Thorac Cardiovasc Surg 92: 972–976

100. Chin A, Fogarty T (1988) Specialized techniques of angioscopic valvulotomy for in situ vein bypass. In: White G, White R (eds) Angioscopy: vascular and coronary applications. Year Book, Chicago

101. Chin A, Fogarty T (1988) Computerized digital angioscopy. In: White G, White R (eds) Angioscopy: vascular and coronary applications. Year Book, Chicago

102. Choy D, Sterzer S, Myler R (1984) Human coronary laser recanalization. Clin Cardiol 7: 377–381

103. Clarke R, Isner J (1985) The use of optical fibers to deliver excimer laser energy to cardiovascular tissue sites. Circulation 72 [Suppl III]: 402

104. Classen M, Dancygier H, Gürtler L, Deinhardt F (1988) Risk of transmitting HIV by endoscopes. Endoscopy 20: 128

105. Conti CR (1977) Coronary arteriography. Circulation 55: 227–237

106. Cortis B, Hussein H, Khandekar C, Pricipe J, Tkaczuk R (1984) Angioscopy in vivo. Cath Cardiovasc Diagn 10: 493–500

107. Cothren R, Hayes C, Kramer J, Sacks B, Kittrell C, Feld M (1986) A multifiber catheter with an optical shield for laser angiosurgery. Lasers Life Sci 1: 1–12

108. Cragg AH, Lund G, Rysavy JA, Salomonowitz E, Castaneda-Zuniga WR, Amplatz K (1984) Percutaneous arterial grafting. Radiology 150: 45–49

109. Cragg A, Lund G, Rysavy J, Castaneda R, Castaneda-Zuniga W, Amplatz K (1983) Nonsurgical placement of arterial endoprosthesis: a new technique using nitinol wire. Radiology 147: 261–263

110. Crispin H (1987) Experience with the vascular brush. J Cardiovasc Surg 28: 48–49
111. Crispin H, van Baarle A (1973) Intravascular observation and surgery using the flexible fibrescope. Lancet 1: 750–751
112. Cumberland D, Tayler D, Procter A (1986) Use of lasers in percutaneous peripheral angioplasty. Semin Intervent Radiol 3: 65–68
113. Cumberland D, Belli A, Myler R, Stertzer S, Crew J (1989) Combined laser/thermal recanalization of peripheral artery occlusions. J Am Coll Cardiol 13 (2): 13A
114. Dacie JE, Lumley JSP (1985) Gortex graft – external carotid artery anastomotic stricture treated by percutaneous transluminal angioplasty. Cardiovasc Intervent Radiol 8: 191–194
115. D'Amelio F, DeLisi S, Rega A (1985) Fiberoptic angioscopes. Opt Eng 24: 672–675
116. Damuth HD Jr, Diamond AB, Rappoport AS (1983) Angioplasty of subclavian artery stenosis proximal to the vertebral origin. AJNR 4: 1239–1245
117. Deckelbaum L, Lam J, Cabin H, Clubb K, Long M (1987) Discrimination of normal and atherosclerotic aorta by laser induced fluorescence. Lasers Surg Med 7: 330–333
118. Deckelbaum L, Sarembock I, Stetz M, O'Brien M, Cutruzzola F, Gmitro A, Ezekowitz M (1988) In-vivo fluorescence spectroscopy of normal and atherosclerotic arteries. J Am Coll Cardiol 11 (2): 173A
119. Dee P, Crosby I (1977) Fibreoptic studies of the aortic valve in dogs. Br Heart J 39: 459–461
120. Demopulos P, Olin E, Wendel Yee G, Kernoff R, Fischell T, Ginsburg R (1988) Balloon angioplasty and rotational tip (Kensey) atherectomy catheter in the rabbit model of atherosclerosis: acute and chronic results. J Am Coll Cardiol 11 (2): 108A
121. de Swart J, El Gamal M, van Gelder L, Michels H, van Ommen G, Baer F (1988) A new technique for angioplasty of occluded coronary arteries not associated with acute myocardial infarction. Eur Heart J 9 [Suppl 1]: 56
122. Dietz U, Pannen B, Erbel R, Haude M, Nixdorff U, Iversen S, Meyer J (1989) Angiographische und histologische Befunde bei der koronaren Hochfrequenzrotationsatherektomie in vitro. Z Kardiol 78 [Suppl I]: 104
123. Dörschel K, Biamino G, Brodzinski T, Axel J, Müller G (1988) Comparison of the feasibility of laserangioplasty using heater probes (HP), sapphire tip (ST) and bare fibres (BF). Eur Heart J 9 [Suppl 1]: 331
124. Doppman JL, Chiro G, Ommaya A (1968) Obliteration of spinal cord arteriovenous malformation by percutaneous embolization. Lancet 2: 47
125. Dorros G, Sachdev N, Lewin R, Mathiak L (1989) The acute outcome of atherectomy in peripheral arterial obstructive disease. J Am Coll Cardiol 13 (2): 108A
126. Dotter C, Buschmann R, McKinney M, Rösch J (1983) Transluminal expandable nitinol coils stent grafting: preliminary report. Radiology 147: 259–260
127. Dotter C (1969) Transluminally placed coilspring endarterial tube grafts: long term patency in canine popliteal artery. Invest Radiol 4: 327–331
128. Dotter C, Judkins M (1964) Transluminal treatment of arteriosclerotic obstruction: description of a new technique and a preliminary of its application. Circulation 30: 654–667
129. Dotter CT, Rösch J, Seaman AJ (1974) Selective clot lysis with low-dose streptokinase. Radiologie 111: 31
130. Dotter CT, Grüntzig A, Schoop, Zeitler E (1983) Percutaneous transluminal angioplasty. Early and late results. Springer, Berlin Heidelberg New York
131. Dunkerly R, Cromer M, Edminton C (1977) Practical techniques for adequate cleaning of endoscopes: a bacteriological study of pHisoHex and Betadine Gastrointest. Endoscopy 23: 148–149
132. Duprat G, Wright K, Charnsangavej C, Wallace S, Gianturco C (1987) Self expanding metallic stens for small vessels: an experimental evaluation. Radiology 162: 469–472

133. Duprat C Jr, Wright K, Charnsangavej C, Wallace S, Gianturco C (1987) Flexible balloon-expanded stent for small vessels. Radiology 162: 276–280
134. Dutto U (1986) Fotografie del systema arterioso ottenute coi raggi Röntgen. Atti Reale Accad Lincei, Serie quinta. Rendiconti ii: 129–31
135. Erbel R, Dietz U, Auth D, Haude M, Nixdorf U, Meyer J (1989) Percutaneous transluminal coronary rotablation during heart catheterization. J Am Coll Cardiol 13 (2): 228A
136. Evans AT (1954) Renal arteriography. AJR 72: 574–580
137. Ferris E, Ledor K, Ben-Avi D, Baker M, Robbins K, McCowan T, Sharma B (1985) Percutaneous angioscopy. Radiology 157: 319–322
138. Ferris E, Ledor K, Baker M (1984) Vascular endoscopy and laser angioplasty in perspective. Appl Radiol 13: 77–82
139. Fischer M (1987) Möglichkeiten und Grenzen der lokalen Thrombolyse peripherer arterieller Verschlüsse. Med Klin 82: 255–258
140. Fleisher H, Thompson B, McCowan T (1986) Angioscopically monitored saphenous vein valvulotomy. J Vasc Surg 4: 360–364
141. Fogarty T, Cranley J, Kraude R (1963) A method for extraction of arterial emboli and thrombi. Surg Gynecol Obstet 116: 241–242
142. Ford KK, Braun SD, Moore E Jr (1985) Percutaneous transluminal angioplasty in diabetic patients: an effective treatment modality. Radiology 155: 852–855
143. Forrester J, Jakubowski A, Hickey A, Litvack F, Grundfest W (1989) Coronary and peripheral vascular angioscopy. In: Vogel J, King S (eds) Interventional cardiology: future directions. Mosby, St. Louis, pp 36–53
144. Forrester J, Litvack F, Grundfest W (1986) Laser angioplasty in cardiovascular disease. Am J Cardiol 57: 990–992
145. Forrester J, Litvack F, Grundfest W, Mohr F, Papaioannou T, Goldenberg T, Laudenslager J (1988) The excimer laser-current knowledge and future prospects. J Intervent Cardiol 1 (1): 75–80
146. Forrester J, Grundfest W, Litvack F, Lee M, Chaux A, Matloff J, Carroll R, Foran R, Berci G, Morgenstern L (1984) Intraoperative vascular endoscopy using flexible fibreoptics. Circulation 70 [Suppl II]: 297
147. Forrester J, Litvack F, Grundfest W, Hickey A (1987) A perspective of coronary disease seen through the arteries of living man. Circulation 75: 505–513
148. Fourrier L, Mordon S, Brunetaud J, Marache P, Lablanche J, Bertrand M (1988) Laser angioplasty of peripheral arteries with a sapphire tip catheter. In: Biamino G, Müller G (eds) Advances in laser medicine I. First German symposium on laser angioplasty. ecomed, Landsberg
149. Fourrier J (1988) Histopathology after rotational angioplasty of peripheral arteries in human beings. J Am Coll Cardiol 11 (2): 109A
150. Fourrier J, Brunetaud J, Prat A, Marache P, Lablanche J, Bertrand M (1987) Percutaneous laser angioplasty with sapphire tip. Lancet 1: 105
151. Frädrich G, Beck A, Bonzel T, Schlosser V (1987) Acute surgical intervention for complications of percutaneous transluminal angioplasty. Eur J Vasc Surg 1: 197–203
152. Frank U, Daschner F (1989) Stellungnahme zur Empfehlung des deutschsprachigen Arbeitskreises für Krankenhaushygiene zum Thema Hygienemaßnahmen bei der Endoskopie. Internist (Berlin) 5: 82–85
153. Freeman I, Isner J, Cal D, Friedman C, Alliger H, Grunwald A (1989) Ultrasonic angioplasty using a new flexible wire system. J Am Coll Cardiol 13 (2): 4A
154. Freitag G, Freitag J, Koch RD (1984) Perkutane transluminale Angioplastik von Karotisstenosen. ROFO 140: 209–212
155. Frommhold W, Gerhard P (1984) Degenerative arterielle Gefäßerkrankungen. Thieme, Stuttgart
156. Gamble W, Ennis R (1967) Experimental intracardiac visualization. N Engl J Med 276: 1397–1403

157. Gardiner GA Jr, Meyerovitz MF, Harrington DP (1985) Dissection complication angioplasty. AJR 145: 627–634
158. Gehani A, Ashley S, Brooks S, Kester R, Ball S, Rees M (1988) Percutaneous angioscopy and sapphire tip lasing of intimal flaps following angioplasty. Heart Vessels 4: 52
159. Geschwind H, Murphy-Chutorian D, Poirot G, Boussignac G, Dubois-Randé J, Mok W (1988) Percutaneous pulsed laser angioplasty guided by spectroscopy. Heart Vessels 4: 52
160. Geschwind H, Fabre M, Chaitman B, Lefebre-Villardebo M, Ladouch A, Boussignac G, Blair J, Kennedy H (1986) Histopathology after Nd: YAG laser percutaneous transluminal angioplasty of peripheral arteries. J Am Coll Cardiol 8: 1089–1095
161. Gilsbach J, Seeger W (1977) Embolisation in der Neurochirurgie. Radiologe 17: 514–520
162. Goar F, Ginsberg R, Mehigan J, Alderman E, Popp R (1990) Intravascular ultrasound evaluation of interventional procedures: comparison with fibreoptic angioscopy. J Am Coll Cardiol 15 (2): 254A
163. Golden DA, Ring EJ, McLean GK, Freiman DB (1982) Percutaneous transluminal angioplasty in the treatment of abdominal angina. AJR 139: 247–249
164. Goldman ML, Land WC, Bradley EL, Anderson J (1976) Transcatheter therapeutic embolization in the management of massive upper gastrointestinal bleeding. Radiology 120: 513–520
165. Gooding GAW, Effeney DJ (1982) Static and real time B-mode sonography of arterial occlusions. AJR 139: 949–953
166. Goodwin WE, Scardino PL, Scott WW (1950) Translumbar aortic puncture and retrograde catherization of the aorta in aortography and renal arteriography. Ann Surg 132: 944–958
167. Graham S, Brands D, Savakus A, Hodgson J (1989) Utility of an intravascular ultrasound imaging device for arterial wall definition and atherectomy guidance. J Am Coll Cardiol 13 (2): 222A
168. Graham D, Smith J, Schwartz J (1986) Endoscopic television: traditional and video endoscopy. Gastrointest Endosc 32: 49–51
169. Greeenstone S, Shore J, Heringman E (1966) Arterial endoscopy (arterioscopy). Arch Surg 93: 811–812
170. Groitl H, Willital G, Meier H, Krebs C (1979) Intraoperative Endoskopie bei Ösophagus- und Analatresien. Z Kinderchir 27 [Suppl]: 116–119
171. Grote R, Freyschmidt J, Walterbusch G (1983) Die perkutane transluminale Angioplastik (PTA) von proximalen Subclaviastenosen. ROFO 138: 660–664
172. Grüntzig A, Hopff H (1974) Perkutane Rekanalisation chronischer arterieller Verschlüsse mit einem neuen Dilatationskatheter. Modifikation der Dottertechnik. Dtsch Med Wochenschr 99: 2502–2510
173. Grüntzig A (1978) Transluminal dilatation of coronary – artery stenosis. Lancet ii: 263–267
174. Grützmacher P, Bussmann WD (1986) Transluminale Dilatation und andere nicht-operative Kathetertechniken in der Behandlung der renovasculären Hypertonie. Klin Wochenschr 64: 884–888
175. Grundfest W, Litvack F, Glick D, Segalowitz J, Treiman R, Cohen L, Foran R, Levin P, Cossman D, Caroll R, Spigelman A, Forrester J (1988) Intraoperative decisions based on angioscopy in peripheral vascular surgery. Circulation 78 [Suppl III]: 1–13
176. Grundfest W, Litvack F, Sherman T (1986) Definition of new pathophysiologic mechanisms and altered decisions: an outcome of intravascular angioscopy. J Am Coll Cardiol 7: 153A
177. Grundfest W, Litvack F, Lee M, Matloff J, Carroll R, Foran R, Berci G, Morgenstern L, Forrester J (1987) The current status of angioscopy and laser angioplasty. J Vasc Surg 5: 667–673

178. Grundfest W, Litvack F, Sherman T, Carroll R, Lee M, Chaux A, Kass R, Matloff J, Berci G, Swan H, Morgenstern L, Forrester J (1985) Delineation of peripheral and coronary detail by intraoperative angioscopy. Ann Surg 202: 394–400

179. Grundfest WS, Litvack F, Sherman T, Carroll R, Lee M, Chaux A (1983) Delineation of peripheral and coronary detail by intraoperative angioscopy. Radiology 148: 161–166

180. Guthaner DF, Schmitz L (1982) Percutaneous transluminal angioplasty of radiation – induced arterial stenoses. Radiology 144: 77–78

181. Hamm C, Kupper W, Schofer J, Mathey D, Bleifeld W (1988) Recanalization of total coronary occlusions with a new catheter system. Eur Heart J 19 [Suppl 1]: 57

182. Haschek E, Lindenthal OT (1896) Ein Beitrag zur praktischen Verwertung der Photographie nach Röntgen. Wien Klin Wochenschr 9: 63–64

183. Hashizume M, Yang Y, Galt S (1987) Intimal response of saphenous vein to intraluminal trauma by simulated angioscopic insertion. J Vasc Surg 5: 862–868

184. Hassenstein S, Haase K, Wehrmann M, Walz R, Karsch K (1989) In vitro Untersuchung über Effekte der Hochfrequenzangioplastie auf atherosklerotisch veränderte Gefäßwand. Z Kardiol 78 [Suppl I]: 20

185. Hasso AN, Bird CR, Zinke DE (1986) Fibromuscular dysplasia of the internal carotid artery: percutaneous transluminal angioplasty. AJR 126: 955–957

186. Heintzen M, Neubaur T, Köhler M, Strauer B (1988) Laser angioplasty of iliac artery stenoses. Heart Vessels 4: 53

187. Heldman D, Mallery J, Spears G, Gessert J, Griffith J, Tobis J, Henry W (1989) Intravascular ultrasound imaging catheter accurately measure area of stenotic aortic valves in vitro. J Am Coll Cardiol 13 (2): 49A

188. Heimworth JA, McGuire J, Felson B (1950) Arteriography of the aorta and its branches by means of the polyethylene catheter. AJR 64: 196–213

189. Hess H, Mietaschk A, Ingrisch H (1982) Kombination der perkutanen transluminalen Angioplastie mit lokaler Thrombolyse. Vasa 11: 282–286

190. Hess H (1986) Zur Entwicklung der thrombolytischen Behandlung des peripheren arteriellen Verschlusses. Vasa 15: 324–327

191. Hess H, Mietaschk A, Brückl R (1987) Peripheral arterial occlusions: a 6 year experience with local low-dose thrombolytic therapy. Radiology 163: 753–757

192. Hickey A, Litvack F, Grundfest W, Lee M, Chaux A, Blanche C, Kass R, Sherntan T, Glick D, Swan H, Matloff J, Forrester J (1987) Coronary angioscopy: the spectrum of disease in the first 100 patients. J Am Coll Cardiol 9 (2): 197A

193. Hirschowitz B, Curtiss L, Peters C, Pollard H (1958) Demonstration of a new gastroscope, the "fibrescope". Gastroenterology 35 (1): 50–52

194. Höfling B, Backa D, Lauterjung L, von Pölnitz A, von Antim T, Jauch K, Simpson J (1988) Percutaneous removal of atheromatous plaques in peripheral arteries. Lancet 2: 384–386

195. Höfling B, Simpson J, Remberger K, Lauterjung L, Backa D (1987) Percutaneous atherectomy in iliac, femoral and popliteal arteries. Klin Wochenschr 65: 58

196. Höfling B, Simpson J, Backa D (1987) Perkutane transluminale Exzision von okkludierendem Plaquematerial (Atherektomie) mit einem neuen Katheter. Z Herz Thorax Gefäßchir 1: 124–129

197. Höfling B, Backa D, Stäblein A, Remberger K, Lauterjung L, Martin E (1987) Erste Erfahrungen mit dem Atherektomie-Katheter. Z Kardiol 76 [Suppl I]: 51

198. Höher M, Hombach V, Hopp H, Hannekum A, Hilger H, Kirche H (1987) Percutaneous and intraoperative coronary angioscopy. Circulation [Suppl IV]: 185

199. Höher M, Hombach V, Hannekum A, Eggeling T, Höpp H, Hilger H (1987) Perkutane und intraoperative Koronarendoskopie. Z Kardiol 76 [Suppl 2]: 21

200. Höher M, Hombach V, Höpp H, Hilger H (1988) Percutaneous coronary angioscopy during cardiac catheterization. J Am Coll Cardiol 11 [Suppl II]: 65A

201. Höher M, Hombach V, Höpp H, Eggeling T, Kochs M, Arnold G, Hannekum A, Hügel W (1988) Diagnostische Bedeutung der Angioskopie bei Patienten mit koronarer Herzkrankheit. Z Kardiol 77: 152–159

202. Höher M, Behrenbeck D, Winter U, Hombach V, Hilger H (1985) Perkutane Gefäßendoskopie mittels ultradünner Fiberendoskope: erste Erfahrungen. Z Kardiol 74 [Suppl III]: 99
203. Höher M, Kochs M, Eggeling T, Haerer W, Hombach V (1990) Verbesserung der Koronarangioskopie durch Anwendung eines Spülkatheters. Z Kardiol 79 [Suppl 1]: 109
204. Höpner F (1979) Kinderchirurgische Indikationen zur Endoskopie des Ösophagus. Z Kinderchir 27 [Suppl]: 54–58
205. Hoffmann MA, Fallon JT, Greenfield AJ (1981) Arterial pathology after percutaneous transluminal angioplasty. AJR 137: 147–156
206. Hombach V, Höher M, Hannekum A, Hügel W, Buran B, Höpp H, Hirche H (1986) Erste klinische Erfahrungen mit der Koronarendoskopie. Dtsch Med Wochenschr 111: 1135–1140
207. Hoyos JM, del Campo CG (1948) Angiography of the thoracic aorta and coronary vessels. Radiology 50: 211–215
208. Huppert P, Duda S, Haase K, Karsch K, Claussen C (1990) Excimer-Laser Angioplastie. Teil II: erste klinische Erfahrungen bei peripherer arterieller Verschlußkrankheit. ROFO 152 (3): 259–263
209. Ichikawa T (1938) Schatten der Nierenarterie, meine Methode zur röntgenologischen Darstellung der Nierenarterie. Z Uro 32: 563–564
210. Inoue K, Kuwaki K, Ueda K (1987) Angioscopy guided coronary thrombolysis. J Am Coll Cardiol 9: 62A
211. Inoue K, Kuwaki K, Takahashi M (1983) Transluminal cardioangioscopy. Circulation 68 [Suppl III]: 7
212. Inoue K, Kuwaki K (1986) In vivo angioscopic demonstration of thrombus as a cause of cyclic flow variation in stenosed canine coronary artery. J Am Coll Cardiol 7: 55–59
213. Inoue K, Kuwaki K, Ochai H, Ueda K, Takano E, Minato H (1989) Percutaneous transluminal coronary angioscopy as the guiding therapy for intracoronary thrombolysis and angioplasty. In: Vogel J, King S (eds) Interventional cardiology: future directions. Mosby, St. Louis, pp 1– 27
214. Inoue K, Kuwaki K, Ueda K, Takano E (1988) Angioscopic macropathology of coronary atherosclerosis in unstable angina and acute myocardial infarction. J Am Coll Cardiol 11 (2): 65A
215. Inoue K, Kuwaki K, Takahashi M (1984) In vivo transluminal angioscopy. Circulation 70 [Suppl II]: 322
216. Ischinger T, Coppenrath K, Weber H, Pesarini A (1990) Ergebnisse und angioskopische Befunde nach Excimer-Laserangioplastie: Laser- oder "Dotter"-Effekte? Z Kardiol 79 [Suppl 1]: 125
217. Itoh T, Hori M (1983) Vascular endoscopy for major vascular reconstruction: experimental and clinical studies. Surgery 93: 391–396
218. Jäger K (1989) Neuere diagnostische Methoden zur nichtinvasiven Lokalisation und hämodynamischen Beurteilung arterieller Obstruktionen. Internist (Berlin) 30: 397–405
219. Jönsson G (1948) Visualization of the coronary arteries. Acta Radiol 29: 536–538
220. Jönsson G (1949) Thoracic aortography by means of a cannula inserted percutaneously into the common carotid artery. Acta Radiol 31: 376–378
221. Kachel R, Endert G, Basche S, Grossmann K, Glaser FH (1987) Percutaneous transluminal angioplasty (dilatation) of carotid, vertebral and innominate artery stenoses. Cardiovasc Intervent Radiol 10: 142–146
222. Kaltenbach M, Vallbracht C (1988) Low speed rotational angioplasty for reopening of chronic artery occlusions – preliminary results. Eur Heart J 9 [Suppl 1]: 56
223. Kandyba J, Burger W, Hartmann A, Niemöller E, Keul H, Sievert H, Schneider M, Kober G (1990) Angiographischer und histologischer Verlauf nach Implantation von Gefäßprothesen (stents) in die Koronararterien gesunder Mini-Schweine. Z Kardiol 79 [Suppl 1]: 22

224. Kappenberger L, Goebel N, Hinterauer L, Tartini R, Steinbrunn W (1982) Stufen-weise Koronardilatation (PTCA) mit Doppelballonkatheter. ROFO 137: 627–631

225. Karsch K, Haase K, Voelker W, Mauser M, Seipel L (1990) Percutaneous coronary excimer laser angioplasty in patients with stable and unstable angina pectoris. J Am Coll Cardiol 15 (2): 245A

226. Katzen BT, Rossi P, Passariello R, Simonetti G (1981) Low dose streptokinase in the treatment of arterial occlusions. AJR 136: 1171–1178

227. Katzen BT (1984) Percutaneous transluminal angioplasty for arterial disease of the lower extremities. AJR 142: 23–26

228. Katzir A (1988) Silver halide optical fibers for endoscopic therapy and diagnosis. Heart Vessels 4: 63

229. Kauffmann GW, Roeren T, Beck A (1985) Verbesserung arteriographischer Techniken durch neue dünne Katheter. Radiologe 25: 48–49

230. Kelling C (1901) Über die Besichtigung der Speiseröhre und des Magens mit biegsamen Instrumenten. Verh Dtsch Naturforsch Arzte 73: 11

231. Kensey K, Nash I, Abrahams C, Lake K, Zarins C (1986) Recanalization of obstructed arteries using a flexible rotating tip catheter. Circulation 74 [Suppl II]: 457

232. Kinney TB, Chin AK, Rurik GW, Finn JC, Shorr PM, Hayden WG, Fogarty TJ (1984) Transluminal angioplasty a mechanical-pathophysiological correlation of its physical mechanisms. Radiology 153: 85–87

233. Klepzig M, Neubaur T, Richter E, Zeitler E, Strauer B (1987) Transfemorale periphere Laserangioplastie. Dtsch Med Wochenschr 112: 324–334

234. Kondos G, Rich S, Levitsky S (1984) Flexible fiberoptic pericardioscopy for the diagnosis of pericardial disease. Circulation 70 [Suppl II]: 322

235. Kozarek R (1987) Direct cholangioscopy and pancreaticoscopy at time of endoscopic cholangiopancreaticography. Am J Gastroenterol 83: 55–59

236. Kozarek R (1988) The future of invasive pancreatico-biliary endoscopy. J Clin Gastroenterol 10: 253–256

237. Krause A, Chapman R, Bigelow J, Salomon N, Okies J, Page U (1983) Early experience with the intraluminal graft prosthesis. Am J Surg 145: 619–622

238. Krepel VM, van Andel GJ, van Erp WFM, Breslau PJ (1985) Percutaneous transluminal angioplasty of the femoropopliteal artery: initial and long term results. Radiology 156: 325–330

239. Kuhl W (1990) Technik und klinische Ergebnisse der Angioskopie im Rahmen einer peripheren Gefäßoperation. Thesis, University of Frankfurt (M)

240. Kumpe DA (1981) Percutaneous dilatation of an abdominal aortic stenosis: three-balloon-catheter technique. Radiology 141: 536–537

241. Kussmaul A (1868) Über Magenspiegelung. Ber Dtsch Natur Ges 112

242. Kuwaki K, Inoue K, Ueda K (1987) Percutaneous transluminal coronary angioscopy during cardiac catheterization: the results of experiences in the first 30 patients. Circulation 76 [Suppl IV]: 186

243. Laerum F, Castaneda Zuniga WR, Rysavy JA, Moore R, Amplatz K (1982) The site of arterial wall rupture in transluminal angioplasty: an experimental study. Radiology 144: 769–770

244. Lammer J, Pilger E, Ascher P, Schmid-Kloiber H (1988) Angioscopy in laser angioplasty of peripheral arteries. Heart Vessels 4: 55

245. Lamerton A (1986) PTA. Br J Surg 73: 91–97

246. Ledor K, Ferris E, ben-Avi D (1985) Percutaneous angioscopy: methodological considerations. Opt Eng 24: 681–682

247. Lee M, Reis R, Lee G, Chan M, Theis J, Ikeda R, Rink J, Petersen L, Solomon B, Siegal R, Hannah H, Hanna E, Bommer W, Mason D (1986) Intraoperative cardiovascular endoscopy in patients with heart disease. Clin Res 33: 12A

248. Lee G, Garcia HJ, Corso P, Chan M, Ring J, Pichard A, Lee K, Reis R, Mason D (1986) Correlation of coronary angioscopic to angiographic findings in coronary artery disease. Am J Cardiol 58: 238–241

249. Lennert K (1987) Technique and results of intraoperative choledochoscopy. Surg Endosc 1: 51–54
250. Léon M, Virmani R, Lenhard S, Almagor Y, Bartorelli A, Prevosti L (1989) Chronic endovascular responses after stent implantation in vein grafts. J Am Coll Cardiol 13 (2): 106A
251. Leuschner U, Hellstern A, Birkenfeld G, Gatzen M, Fischer H, Leuschner M, Kurtz W, Wendt T (1987) Methyl-*tert*-butyl-ether (MTBE) in problem cases: gallbladder endoscopy for treatment assessment. Gastroenterology 92 (5): 1750
252. Leuschner U, Hellstern A, Wendt T, Birkenfeld G, Leuschner M, Gatzen M, Kurtz W, Fischer H (1988) Endoscopy of the gallbladder as control of gallstone therapy with methyl-*tert*-butyl-ether. Am J Gastroenterol 83 (2): 169–172
253. Likungu J, Grube E, Kirchhoff P, Quade G, Schubert W (1987) Intraoperative Darstellung der Koronararterien mit hochfrequentem Ultraschall vor und nach Revascularisation. Herz Kreisl 19: 199–202
254. Lindgren E (1953) Technique of abdominal aortography. Acta Radiol 39: 205
255. Litvack F, Grundfest W, Hickey A, Lee D, Chaux A, Forrester J (1987) Coronary angioscopy: correlation of morphology with clinical syndrome. Eur Heart J 8 [Suppl II]: 222
256. Litvack F, Grundfest W, Mohr F, Strul B, Goldenberg T, Roth F, Kirchhoff P, Forrester J (1988) Percutaneous "hot tip" angioplasty in man by radio frequency catheter system. J Am Coll Cardiol 11 (2): 108A
257. Litvack F, Grundfest W, Lee M, Carroll R, Foran R, Chaux A, Berci G, Rose H, Matloff J, Forrester J (1985) Angioscopic visualization of blood vessel interior in animals and humans. Clin Cardiol 8: 65–70
258. Litvack F, Hickey A, Grundfest W, Lee M, Sherman T, Doyle L, Chaux A, Blanche C, Kass R, Matloff J, Swan H, Forrester J (1986) Angioscopy is superior to angiography for detecting complex atheroma. Circulation 74 [Suppl II]: 362
259. Löhr E, Budach V, Birkner P, Hartjes H, Spira G, Weichert HC (1983) PTA der Nierenarterien – ein therapeutisches Prinzip zur nichtoperativen Behandlung einer durch Nierenarterienstenose ausgelösten Hypertonie. Radiologe 23: 215–220
260. Loening K, Sitieda A (1910) Die Untersuchung des Magens mit dem Magenspiegel. Mitt Grenzgeb Med Chir 21: 181
261. Lu CT, Zarins CK, Yang CF, Turcotte JK (1982) Long-segment arterial occlusion: percutaneous transluminal angioplasty. AJR 138: 119–121
262. Maas D, Zollikofer C, Largiadere F, Senning A (1984) Radiological follow-up of transluminally inserted vascular endoprosthesis: an experimental study using expanding spirals. Radiology 152: 659–663
263. Maaßen W (1989) Thorakoskopie: chirurgische Technik. Pneumologie 43: 53–54
264. Maisch B, Ertl G, Drude L, Kochsiek K (1988) Pericardioscopy of effusions – technique and future implications. Eur Heart J 9 [Suppl A]: 195
265. Maisch B, Drude L (1989) Perikardioskopie bei Perikarderguß. Z Kardiol 78 [Suppl 4]: 37
266. Manegold B, Joppich I (1979) Laparoskopie und endoskopische retrograde Cholangiopancreaticographie (ERCP) im Kindesalter. Z Kinderchir 27 [Suppl]: 125–133
267. Martin EC, Fankuchen EI, Karlson KB (1981) Angioplasty for femoral artery occlusion: comparison with surgery. AJR 137: 915–917
268. Mathias K, Bockenheimer S, von Reuttern G, Heiss HW, Ostheim-Dzerowycz W (1983) Katheterdilatation hirnversorgender Arterien. Radiologe 23: 208–214
269. Matsumoto T, Koyanagi N, Hashizume M, Yang Y, DuPree J, Maitra S (1989) Angioscopy and intimal response. In: White G, White R (eds) Angioscopy: vascular and coronary applications. Year Book Medical Publishers, Chicago
270. Matsumoto T, Hashizume M, Yang Y (1987) Direct vision valvulotomy in in situ venous bypass. Surg Gynecol Obstet 165: 362–364
271. Matsumoto A, Teitelbaum G, Barth K, Carvlin M, Savin M, Strecker E (1989) Tantalum vascular stents: in vivo evaluation with MR imaging. Radiology 170: 753–755

272. Mazieres M (1987) L'endoprothèse coronarienne: sera-t-elle la solution au problème des restenoses après angioplastie coronaire? Panorama Med 14: 2517
273. McCowan T, McAlister M, Ferris E (1988) Angioscopic evaluation of vascular anastomoses of the lower extremities in the canine model. J Arlzansas Med Soc 84: 373-376
274. McCowan T, Robbins K, Uthman E (1985) Angioscopic monitoring of in vivo laser angioplasty. SPIE Opt Fibers Med Biol 576: 39-41
275. Mehigan J, Olcoll C (1986) Video angioscopy as an alternative to intraoperative arteriography. Am J Surg 152: 139-145
276. Mehigan J (1989) Angioscopic preparation of the in situ saphenous vein for arterial bypass: technical considerations. In: White G, White R (eds) Angioscopy: vascular and coronary applications. Year Book, Chicago
277. Miller R (1986) Endoscopic instrumentation: evolution, physical principles and clinical aspects. Br Med Bull 42: 223-226
278. Mizuno K, Arakawa K, Shibuya T, Horiuchi K, Okamoto Y, Miyamoto A, Isojima K, Kurita A, Satomura K, Nakamura H, Arai T, Kikuchi M (1988) A serial observation of coronary thrombosis in vivo by a new angioscope. J Am Coll Cardiol 11 [Suppl II]: 30A
279. Mizuno K, Miyamoto A, Satomura K, Shibuya T, Okamoto Y, Seguchi H, Isojima K, Kurita A, Arai T, Nakamura H (1989) Angioscopic endothelial macropathology in patients with acute coronary syndromes. J Am Coll Cardiol 13 (2): 14A
280. Moniz E (1927) L'encéphalographie artérielle, son importance dans la localisation des tumeurs cérébrales. Rev Neurol (Paris) 11: 73
281. Moosdorf R, Scheid H, Stertmann W, Hehrlein W (1987) Koronare Endoskopie – eine neue intraoperative Kontrollmethode nach Endarteriektomie der rechten Kranzarterie. Thorac Cardiovasc Surg 35 [Suppl 1]: 14-15
282. Morice M, Marco J, Castillo-Fenoy A, Fajadet J, Glatt B, Royer T (1988) A new technique for investigation and treatment of acute myocardial infarction: percutaneous coronary angioscopy. Eur Heart J 9 [Suppl A]: 211
283. Morice M, Marco J, Fajadet J (1987) Percutaneous coronary angioscopy before and after angioplasty in acute myocardial infarction. Preliminary results. Circulation 76 [Suppl IV]: 282
284. Moser K, Shure D, Harell J, Tulumello J (1980) Angioscopic visualization of pulmonary emboli. Chest 77: 198-201
285. Motarjeme A, Keifer JW, Zuska AJ, Nabawi P (1985) Percutaneous transluminal angioplasty for treatment of subclavian steal. Radiology 155: 611-615
286. Müller-Kühlkamp Th (1990) Methodische Aspekte und Anwendungsmöglichkeiten der Angioskopie mit ultradünnen Fiberglasendoskopen. Thesis, University of Frankfurt (M)
287. Murray G (1950) A cardioscope. Angiology 1: 334-336
288. Murray RR Jr, Hewes RC, White RI Jr, Mitchell SE, Auster M, Chang R, Kadir S, Kinnison ML, Kaufman SL (1987) Long-segment femoropopliteal stenoses: is angioplasty a boon or a bust? Radiology 162: 473-477
289. Myler R, Stertzer S, Millhouse F, Crew F, McMorrow J, Hidalgo B (1984) Intravascular angioscopy (IVA) and human peripheral angioplasty. Circulation 70 [Suppl II]: 265
290. Nitsch J (1990) Laserangioplastie und Koronarendoskopie. Endoskopie Heute 1: 13-16
291. Noy M, Harrison L, Holmes G, Cockel R (1980) The significance of bacterial contamination of fibre-optic endoscopes. J Hosp Infect 1: 53-61
292. Nyström B (1987) Sterilisation oder Desinfektion von Endoskopen? Hyg Med 12: 174-175
293. Ödman P (1956) Percutaneous selective angiography of the main branches of the aorta. Acta Radiol 45: 1-14
294. Olcott C (1987) Clinical applications of video angioscopy. J Vasc Surg 5: 664-666
295. Olinger C (1977) Carotid artery endoscopy (autopsy). Surg Neurol 7: 7-13

296. O'Neill W, Bates E, Kirsh M, Bassett J, Sakwa M, Elliot M, Doppke D, Beaumont W (1989) Mechanical transluminal coronary endarterectomy: initial clinical results with the Auth mechanical rotary catheter. J Am Coll Cardiol 13 (2): 227A

297. Palmaz JC, Windeler SA, Garcia F, Tio FO, Sibbitt RR, Reuter SR (1986) Arteriosclerotic rabbit aortas: expandable intraluminal grafting. Radiology 160: 723–725

298. Palmaz J, Sibbitt R, Reuter S, Tio F, Rice W (1985) Expandable intraluminal graft a preliminary study. Radiology 156: 73–77

299. Palmaz J, Sibbitt R, Tio F, Reuter S, Peters J, Garcia F (1985) Expandable intraluminal vascular graft a feasibility study. Surgery 99: 199–205

300. Pandian N, Kreis A, Brockway B, Sacharoff A, Boleza E, Caro R (1989) Detection of intravascular thrombus by high frequency intraluminal ultrasound angioscopy: in vitro and in vivo studies. J Am Coll Cardiol 13 (2): 5A

301. Peirce EC, Ramey WP (1953) Renal arteriography: report of a percutaneous method using the femoral artery approach and a disposable catheter. J Urol 69: 578–585

302. Perez J, Hinohara T, Quigley P, Lee M, Hoffmann P, Mikal E, Phillips H, Stack R (1988) In-vitro and in-vivo experimental results using a new wire guided concentric atherectomy device. J Am Coll Cardiol 11 (2): 109A

303. Peura D, Tranmont E (1987) AIDS: the scope of the problem and the problem of the ‚scope'. Gastrointest Endosc 33: 122–124

304. Pinet F, Archimbaud J, Fredenucci R (1966) Problèmes posés par l'endoscopie cardiovasculaire. Presse Med 74: 2351–2352

305. Prevosti L, Lawrence J, Leon M, Kramer W, Dy L, Smith P, Bonner R (1987) Reduced surface thrombogenicity after thermal ablation in plaque. Circulation 76 [Suppl IV]: 408

306. Probst P, Cerny P, Owens A (1983) Patency after femoral angioplasty: correlation of angiographic appearence with clinical findings. AJR 140: 1227–1233

307. Radner S (1945) An attempt at the roentgenologic visualization of coronary blood vessels in man. Acta Radiol 26: 497–502

308. Radner S (1948) Thoracical aortography by catheterization from the radial artery. Acta Radiol 29: 178–183

309. Ramee S, White C, Banks A, Aita M, Doyle T, Michaels M, Graeber C, Price H (1988) Percutaneous coronary angioscopy using a steerable microangioscope. J Am Coll Cardiol 11 [Suppl II]: 173A

310. Raso AM, Carlin C, Falco E (1986) La valoracion de los troncos supraaorticos por medio de la ultrasonographia Doppler y angioscopio. Angiologia 38: 306–314

311. Richens D, Rees M, Watson D (1987) Laser coronary angioplasty under direct vision. Lancet 2: 683–690

312. Riemann J, Kohler B (1988) Peroral cholangioscopy – an improved method in the diagnosis of common bile duct diseases. Gastroenterology 94: A377

313. Ring EJ, Freiman DB, McLean GK (1982) Percutaneous recanalization of common iliac artery occlusions: an unacceptable complication rate? AJR 139: 587–592

314. Ritchie J, Hansen D, Vracko H. Auth D (1986) In vivo rotational thrombectomy evaluation by angioscopy. Circulation 74 [Suppl II]: 1822

315. Ritter H, Großmann K, Basche S, Heerklotz I, Schiffmann R, Schumann E (1982) Die perkutane transluminale Angioplastik (PTA) von Aortenbogenästen. ROFO 136: 365–370

316. Rizk C, Goodale R, Amplatz K (1973) Vascular endoscopy. Radiology 106: 33–36

317. Rodgers G, Raizner A, Cromeens D, Wright K, Stevens C, Roubin G, Minor S (1989) Coronary spasm induced by stent implantation. J Am Coll Cardiol 13 (2): 194A

318. Romaniuk P, Wierny L, Münster W (1985) Langzeiteffektivität der angioplastischen Therapie iliakaler und femoro-poplitealer Obstruktionen im Vergleich zur Operation. In: Oeser H (ed) Angiologie-Symposium. VEB Gesundheit, Berlin (DDR), pp 39–49

319. Rudolph H, Werner H (1988) Hygienemaßnahmen bei der Endoskopie. Hyg Med 13: 354–356

320. Sanborn T, Rygaard J, Westbrook B, Lazar H, McCormick J, Roberts A (1986) Intraoperative angioscopy of saphenous vein and coronary arteries. J Thorac Cardiovasc Surg 91: 339–343

321. Sanborn T (1986) Vascular endoscopy: current state of the art. Br Med Bull 42: 270–275

322. Santos R dos, Lamas A, Caldas JP (1929) Die Arteriographie der Extremitäten, der Aorta und ihrer abdominalen Äste. ROFO 40: 384

323. Satava R (1987) Comparison of direct and indirect video endoscopy. Gastrointest Endosc 33: 69–72

324. Satava R, Poe W, Joyce G (1988) Current generation video endoscopes. A critical evaluation. Am Surg 54: 73–77

325. Sawton T (1987) Intraoperative angioscopy of saphenous vein and coronary arteries. J Thoracic Cardiovasc Surg 9: 339

326. Schatz R, Palmaz J, Penn I (1989) Balloon expandable intravascular stents (BEIS) in human coronary arteries: a follow-up report. J Am Coll Cardiol 13 (2): 106A

327. Schrempp K, Müller G, Günther D (1980) Komplikationen bei Angiographien. Radiologe 20: 135–140

328. Schwartz A, Aulich A, Lahrkamp H (1986) Percutaneous transluminal angioscopy: a new approach to intravasal interventional techniques. Lasers 1: 5

329. Schwartz A, Aulich A, Lahrkamp H (1987) Percutaneous transluminal angioscopy: a new approach to intravascular interventional techniques. Lasers 3: 30–32

330. Schwartz A, Aulich A (1988) Percutaneous transluminal angioscopy. In: Biamino G, Müller G (eds) Advances in laser medicine I. First German symposium on laser angioplasty. ecomed, Landsberg

331. Seeger J, Abela G (1986) Angioscopy as an adjunct to arterial reconstructive surgery: a preliminary report. J Vasc Surg 4: 315–320

332. Seeliger K (1973) Direkte intravasculare fibroskopische Lymphoskopie und Ductus thoracicus Kanülierung. Folia Angiol 21: 287–292

333. Seldinger SI (1953) Catheter replacement of the needle in percutaneous arteriography: a new technique. Acta Radiol 39: 368–376

334. Shapiro M, Ausländer M, Shapiro M (1987) The electronic video endoscope: clinical experience with 1200 diagnostic and therapeutic cases in the community hospital. Gastrointest Endosc 33: 63–68

335. Sherman C, Litvack F, Grundfest W, Lee M, Chaux A, Kass R, Swan H, Matloff J, Forrester J (1985) Fiberoptic coronary angioscopy identifies thrombus in all patients with unstable angina. Circulation 72 [Suppl II]: 446

336. Sherman C, Litvack F, Grundfest W, Lee M, Hickey A, Chaux A, Kass R, Blanche C, Matloff J, Morgenstern L, Ganz W, Swan H, Forrester J (1986) Coronary angioscopy in patients with unstable angina pectoris. N Engl J Med 315: 913–919

337. Shore J, Berci G (1976) An improved flexible cholangioscope. Endoscopy 8: 41–45

338. Shure D, Moser K, Harrell J, Hartman M (1981) Identification of pulmonary emboli in the dog: comparison of angioscopy and perfusion scanning. Circulation 64: 618–621

339. Shure D, Simmons K (1984) Angioscope 6 ‚sees' chronic pulmonary emboli. J Am Med Assoc 251: 698–699

340. Shure S, Cregoratos C, Mose M (1984) Angioscopy is useful in the evaluation of chronic pulmonary arterial obstruction. Circulation 70 [Suppl II]: 182

341. Simonetti G, Rossi P, Passariello R (1983) Iliac artery rupture: a complication of transluminal angioplasty. AJR 140: 989–922

342. Simpson J, Johnson D, Thapliyal H, Marks D, Braden L (1985) Transluminal atherectomy: a new approach to the treatment of atherosclerotic vascular disease. Circulation 72 [Suppl II]: 141–146

343. Simpson J (1988) Percutaneous coronary atherectomy. J Am Coll Cardiol 11 (2): 110A

344. Simpson J, Blaim D, Robert E, Harrison D (1982) A new catheter system for coronary angioplasty. Am J Cardiol 49: 1216–1222
345. Smalling R, Cassidy D, Schmidt W, Wise G, Felli P, Barrett R, Boseck G (1989) Initial experience with a flexible rotational atherectomy system designed for removal of coronary and small peripheral artery atheromas. J Am Coll Cardiol 13 (2): 223A
346. Sniderman K, Bodner L, Saddekni S, Srur M, Sos T (1984) Percutaneous embolectomy by transcatheter aspiration. Radiology 150: 357–361
347. Sos TA, Pickering TG, Sniderman KW (1984) Percutaneous transluminal renal angioplasty in renovascular hypertension due to atheroma or fibromuscular dysplasia. Radiology 154: 817–818
348. Spears J, Spokojny A, Marais H, Grossman W (1985) Coronary angioscopy during cardiac catheterization. J Am Coll Cardiol 6: 93–97
349. Spears J, Marais H, Serur J (1983) In vivo coronary angioscopy. J Am Coll Cardiol 1: 1311–1314
350. Spears J, Marais H, Serur J, Paulin S, Grossman W (1982) In vivo coronary angioscopy. Circulation 66 [Suppl II]: 366
351. Starck E, McDermott J, Crummy A, Tuntipseed W, Acher C, Burgess J (1985) Percutaneous aspiration thromboembolectomy. Radiology 156: 61–66
352. Strandness D (1986) Ultrasound in the study of atherosclerosis. Ultrasound Med Biol 12: 453–456
353. Strecker E, Romaniuk P, Schneider B, Westphal M, Zeitler E, Wolf H, Freudenberger N (1988) Perkutan implantierbare, durch Ballon aufdehnbare Gefäßprothese: erste klinische Ergebnisse. Dtsch Med Wochenschr 113: 583–542
354. Susawa T, Yui Y, Hattori R (1987) Direct observation of coronary thrombus using a newly developed ultrathin (1.2 mm) flexible angioscope. J Am Coll Cardiol 9: 197A
355. Takahashi M, Yui Y, Susawa T (1987) Evaluation of coronary thrombus by a newly developed ultrathin (0.75 mm) flexible quartz microfiber angioscope. Circulation 76 [Suppl IV]: 282
356. Tanabe T, Yokota A, Sugie S (1980) Cardiovascular fibreoptic endoscopy: development and clinical application. Surgery 87: 375–378
357. Thiele B, Strandness D Jr (1983) Accuracy of angiographic quantification of peripheral atherosclerosis. Prog Cardiovasc Dis 26: 223–236
358. Tillander H (1956) Selective angiography of the abdominal aorta with a guided catheter. Acta Radiol 45: 21–26
359. Tobis J, Mallery J, Mahon D, Griffith J, Gessert J, MacLeay L, McCroe M, Bessen M, Henry W (1989) Intravascular ultrasound visualization of atheroma plaque removal by atherectomy. J Am Coll Cardiol 13 (2): 222A
360. Tomaru T, Uchida Y, Masuo M (1987) Experimental canine arterial thrombus formation and thrombolysis: a fiberoptic study. Am Heart J 114: 69–74
361. Tomaru T, Uchida Y, Sugimoto T (1988) Fiberoptic study on the effects of transluminal angioplasty in experimental occlusive arterial thrombosis. Am Heart J 115: 312–317
362. Totty WG, Gilula LA, McClennan BL, Ahmed P, Sherman LA (1982) Low-dose intervascular fibrinolytic therapy. Radiology 143: 59–69
363. Towne J, Bernhard V (1977) Vascular endoscopy – an adjunct to carotid surgery. Stroke 8: 569–571
364. Towne J, Bernhard V (1977) Vascular endoscopy: useful tool or interesting toy? Surgery 82: 415–419
365. Uchida Y, Masuo M, Tomaru T, Kato A, Sugimoto T (1986) Fiberoptic observation of thrombosis and thrombolysis in isolated human coronary arteries. Am Heart J 4: 691–696
366. Uchida Y, Tomaru T, Nakamura F, Furuse A, Fujimori Y (1987) Percutaneous coronary angioscopy in patients with ischemic heart diseases. Am Heart J 114: 1216
367. Uchida Y, Tomaru T, Kato A (1987) Angioscopy of blood flow through stenotic arteries: rheologic mechanisms of thrombosis. Am Heart J 114: 63–69

368. Uchida Y, Oshima T, Shibuya I (1988) Percutaneous angioscopy of the right side of the heart in humans. CV World Report 1: 13–17
369. Uchida Y, Furuse A, Hasegawa K (1987) Percutaneous coronary angioscopy using a novel balloon guiding catheter in patients with ischemic heart diseases. Circulation 76 [Suppl IV]: 185
370. Uchida Y, Masuo M, Tomaru T, Kato A (1985) Fiberoptic observation of coronary luminal changes caused by coronary angioplasty. Circulation 72 (3): 218
371. Urban P, Sigwart U, Kaufmann U, Kappenberger L (1989) Restenosis within coronary stents: possible effect of previous angioplasty. J Am Coll Cardiol 13 (2): 107A
372. Vallbracht C, Suss B, Awiszus H, Prignitz I, Liermann G, Kollath J, Landgraf H, Schoop W, Kaltenbach M (1988) Low speed rotational angioplasty – acute results and complications in 33 patients with chronic vessel obstruction. Eur Heart J 9 [Suppl 1]: 333
373. van Andel GJ (1975) Transluminale angioplastiek volgens Dotter. Ned Tijdschr Geneeskd 119: 343–344
374. van Stiegman G, Bartle E, Pearce W (1985) Vascular endoscopy with a new laser capable angioscope. Lasers Surg Med 5: 170
375. van Stiegmann G, Pearce W, Bartle E (1987) Flexible angioscopy seems faster and more specific than arteriography. Arch Surg 122: 279–282
376. van Stiegmann G, Khan D, Rose A (1984) Endoscopic laser endarteriectomy. Surg Gynecol Obstet 158: 529–534
377. Vielledent C, Geschwind H, Boussignac G, Gaujour B, Teisseire B (1986) Debris after laser arterial recanalization. Lasers Med Surg 2: 31–34
378. Vincent J (1986) Live cardioscopy, an experimental study. Lasers 1: 5
379. Vincent G, Fox J (1985) Cardiovascular endoscopy. Cardiovasc Rev Rep 6: 1227–1234
380. Vitek JJ, Raynion BC, Oh SJ (1984) Innominate artery angioplasty. AJNR 5: 113–115
381. Voigt K, Goerttler U (1973) Indikationen und Grenzen der verschiedenen angiographischen Methoden zum Nachweis von stenosierenden Prozessen der supraaortischen Arterien. Radiologe 13: 422–428
382. Vollmar J, Junghanns K (1969) Die Arterioskopie. Langenbecks Arch Klin Chir 325: 1201–1212
383. Vollmar J, Storz L (1974) Vascular endoscopy: possibilities and limits of its clinical application. Surg Clin North Am 54: 111–122
384. Vollmar J (1969) Die Gefäßendoskopie. Ein neuer Weg der intraoperativen Gefäßdiagnostik. Endoscopy 1: 141–151
385. Vollmar J, Heyden B, Hamann H (1979) Wertigkeit intraoperativer Kontrollverfahren aus chirurgischer Sicht. In: Hild R, Spaan G (eds). Therapiekontrolle in der Angiologie. Witzstrock, Baden-Baden
386. Vollmar J, Loeprecht H, Hutschenreiter H (1987) Advances in vascular endoscopy. Thorac Cardiovasc Surg 35: 334–341
387. von Pölnitz A, Backa D, Nehrlich C, Hofling B (1989) Histological evaluation of "vessel biopsies" obtained with the Simpson atherectomy catheter. J Am Coll Cardiol 13 (2): 149A
388. Weibull H, Bergqvist D, Jonsson K, Karlsson S, Takolander R (1987) Complications after percutaneous transluminal angioplasty in the iliac, femoral and popliteal arteries. J Vasc Surg 5: 681–686
389. Wendt T, Müller T, Eckel L, Krause E, Rauber K, Riemann H, Sarai C, Satter P, Sievert H, Stauder M, Vallbracht C, Kober G, Kaltenbach M (1987) In vivo Angioskopie: Technik, Indikationen und Ergebnisse beim Menschen. Z Kardiol 76 [Suppl I]: 51
390. Wendt T, Eckel L, Krause E, Müller T, Radünz N, Sarai C, Sievert H, Vallbracht C, Satter P, Kaltenbach M, Kober G (1987) Coronary balloon dilatation – angioscopic findings. Eur Heart J 8 [Suppl II]: 222

391. Wendt T, Reinemer H, Müller T, Panitz H, Friedel M, Schneider M, Hübner K, Kaltenbach M, Kober G (1988) Angioskopie, Angiographie und pathologische Anatomie des Kranzgefäßsystems. Z Kardiol 77 [Suppl 1]: 149
392. Wendt T, Eckel L, Kaltenbach M, Krause E, Müller T, Radünz N, Sarai C, Satter P, Schräder R, Sievert H, Vallbracht C, Kober G (1988) Coronary angioscopy during cardiac catheterization and surgery. In: Reiber J, Serruys P (eds) New developments in quantitative arteriography. Kluwer, Rotterdam
393. Wendt T, Eckel L, Krause E, Müller T, Radünz N, Sarai C, Sievert H, Vallbracht C, Satter P, Kaltenbach M, Kober G (1988) Coronary balloon dilatation – angioscopic findings. In: Biamino G, Müller G (eds) Advances in laser medicine I. VEB Gesundheit, Berlin (DDR)
394. Wendt T, Moosdorf R, Bettinger R, Kamlot A, Reinemer H, Scheld H, Hehrlein F, Kober G (1988) Immediate angioscopic results following human coronary argon laser angioplasty. Heart Vessels 4 (1): 63
395. Wendt T, Moosdorf R, Bettinger R, Kamlot A, Hehrlein W, Kober G (1989) Intraoperative koronare Argon-Laser-Angioplastie: angioskopische und angiographische Ergebnisse. Z Kardiol 78 [Suppl I]: 21
396. Wendt T, Bettinger R, Kober G (1990) Angioskopie der Herzkranzgefäße. Vers Med 42: 83–88
397. Wendt T (1990) Neue Einblicke. Hofmann, Frankfurt
398. Wenz W, (1967) Angiographische Darstellung der Gallenblasenarterien. ROFO 106: 387–392
399. Wenz W, Beduhn D, Roth FJ, van Kaick G, Czembirek H (1970) Abdominale Angiographie: Technik, Pathomorphologie, Indikationen. Rontgenpraxis 23: 97–124
400. Wenz W, van Kaick G, Roth FJ (1974) Abdominal angiography. Springer, Berlin Heidelberg New York
401. Wenz W, Beck A, Richter G, Nöldge G (1988) Angiographie heute. Gockel HP (ed) Jahrbuch der Radiologie 1988. Regensberg and Biermann, Bielefeld, pp 13–27
402. Wenz W (1984) Röntgendiagnostik im Umbruch. Radiologe 24: 1–4
403. White C, White R, Kopchok G (1988) Angioscopic thromboembolectomy: preliminary observations with a recent technique. J Vasc Surg 7: 318–325
404. White G, White R, Kopchok G (1987) Intraoperative video angioscopy compared with arteriography during peripheral vascular operations. J Vasc Surg 6: 488–495
405. White G (1989) Techniques of angioscopy in the peripheral vascular system. In: White G, White R (eds) Angioscopy vascular and coronary applications. Year Book, Chicago
406. Wierny L, Plass R, Porstmann W (1973) Langzeitbeobachtungen nach transluminaler Katheterrekanalisation arterieller Obliterationen nach Dotter und Judkins. Zentralbl Chir 98: 1761–1772
407. Wilms GE, Smits J, Baert AL, Wolf L (1985) Percutaneous transluminal angioplasty in fibromuscular dysplasia of the internal carotid artery: one year clinical and morphological follow-up. Cardiovasc Intervent Radiol 8: 20–23
408. Wolf GL, LeeVeen RF, Ring EJ (1984) Potential mechanism of angioplasty. Cardiovasc Intervent Radiol 7: 11–17
409. Wollenek G, Laufer G, Horvath R, Stangl G, Wolner E (1986) Thermal effects of far ultraviolet excimer laser radiation in vessel walls. Lasers 1: 9
410. Wollenek G, Laufer G, Fasol R, Zilla P, Wolner E (1986) Laser-induced vascular lesions by cw-Nd: YAG and pulsed UV-lasers during angioplastic procedures. Thorac Cardiovasc Surg 34: 63–65
411. Wright K, Wallace S, Charsangavej C, Cianturco C (1985) Percutaneous endovascular stents: an experimental evaluation. Radiology 156: 69–72
412. Yock P, Linker D, Thapliyal H (1988) Real-time, two-dimensional catheter ultrasound: a new technique for high-resolution intravascular imaging. J Am Coll Cardiol 11: 130A

413. Zacca N, Raizner A, Noon G, Short H, Weilbächer D, Gotto A, Roberts R (1988) Short term follow up of patients tested with a recently developed rotational atherectomy device and in vivo assessment of the particles generated. J Am Coll Cardiol 11 (2): 109A
414. Zeitler E (1972) Die perkutane Rekanalisation arterieller Obliterationen mit Katheter nach Dotter (Dotter-Technik). Dtsch Med Wochenschr 97: 1392–1394
415. Zeitler E, Schoop W, Zahnow W (1971) The treatment of occlusive arterial disease by transluminal angioplasty. Radiology 99: 19–26
416. Zeitler E, Richter EI, Roth FJ, Schoop W (1983) Results of percutaneous transluminal angioplasty. Radiology 146: 57–60
417. Zeitler E, Müller R (1969) Erste Ergebnisse mit der Katheterrekanalisation nach Dotter bei arterieller Verschlußkrankheit. ROFO 111: 345–352
418. Zeitler E (1988) Laser-angioplasty and dynamic PTA in comparison to balloon dilatation. In: Biamino G, Müller G (eds) Advances in laser medicine I. First German symposium on laser angioplasty. ecomed, Landsberg
419. Zollikofer C, Largiader I, Bruhlmann W, Uhlschmid G, Marthy A (1988) Endovascular stenting of veins and grafts: preliminary clinical experience. Radiology 167: 707–712
420. Zollikofer CL, Salomonowitz E, Sibley R, Chain J, Bruhlmann WF, Castaneda-Zuniga WR, Amplatz K (1984) Transluminal angioplasty evaluated by electron microscopy. Radiology 153: 369–374
421. Zollikofer CL, Salomonowitz E, Bruhlmann WF, Castaneda-Zuniga WR, Amplatz K (1986) Dehnungs-, Verformungs- und Berstungscharakteristika häufig verwendeter Ballondilatationskatheter. ROFO 144: 40–46

Subject Index

Springer-Verlag
and the Environment

We at Springer-Verlag firmly believe that an international science publisher has a special obligation to the environment, and our corporate policies consistently reflect this conviction.

We also expect our business partners – paper mills, printers, packaging manufacturers, etc. – to commit themselves to using environmentally friendly materials and production processes.

The paper in this book is made from low- or no-chlorine pulp and is acid free, in conformance with international standards for paper permanency.